LIFE WITH CHARLIE

Coping With An Alzheimer Spouse Or Other
Dementia Patient And Keeping Your Sanity

LIFE WITH CHARLIE

Coping With An Alzheimer Spouse Or Other
Dementia Patient And Keeping Your Sanity

By

Carol Heckman-Owen

Pathfinder Publishing of California
Ventura, CA

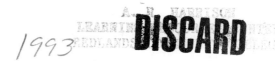

LIFE WITH CHARLIE

By

Carol Heckman-Owen

Published By:
Pathfinder Publishing of California
458 Dorothy Avenue
Ventura, CA 93003
(805) 642-9278

Library of Congress Cataloging-in-Publication Data

Heckman-Owen, Carol
    Life with Charlie : coping with an Alzheimer spouse or other dementia patient and keeping your sanity / by Carol Heckman-Owen.
        p.   cm.
    Includes bibliographical references and index.
    ISBN 0-934793-41-7 : $9.95
        1. Charlie — Mental health. 2. Alzheimer's disease — Patients — United States — Biography. 3. Alzheimer's disease — Patients — Care. 4. Alzheimer's disease — Patients — Family relationships. I. Title.
    RC523.H43   1992
    362.1 ' 96831 ' 0092 — dc20
    (B)   91-38235
                                                                              CIP

ISBN 0-934793-41-7

DEDICATION

To my parents, Herbert and Clara, who, by their example, taught me to love God, life, and to appreciate nature. They inspired me to reach my highest potential.

To my children, Jay, Susan, and Darla for their encouragement and financial assistance.

And, last but not least, to caregivers all over the world, who have struggled or are still struggling with the problems of Alzheimer's or other dementia ailments.

CONTENTS

FOREWORD

This is not just a book about Alzheimer's disease. It is a story of what it means to be human.

Too often in cases of Alzheimer's disease people lose sight of the human beings affected by the illness. Yet the irritable, confused person with Alzheimer's is still a human being, and the struggling, confused caregiver is still a human being.

What I like best about the story of Carol Heckman-Owen and her husband Charlie is the romance and the love. These two high school sweethearts were newlyweds in a brand new marriage when the disease began to affect Charlie's memory and personality. The care and the realism contained in Carol's account are extremely helpful to other families and fascinating to read.

There are several million families affected by the Disease, yet there is a noticeable lack of books by the family members themselves.

I recommend this book to other caregivers as an example of how to do the right thing for an ailing loved one, and how to make sure you stay healthy yourself in the process.

I also recommend it to the doctors, nurses, social workers, researchers, insurance personnel, and others who work with Alzheimer's cases and yet rarely get to see the human side of the illness described with such skill and perspective. I hope this book inspires others as it has ʾspired me.

Leonard Felder, Ph.D.
Author, *When A Loved One Is Ill*

ACKNOWLEDGMENTS

Special appreciation goes:

To my publisher, Eugene Wheeler, who believed in my book and enriched it with his creative suggestions.

To Eugenie Wheeler, who encouraged me when I felt despondent and offered helpful writing suggestions.

To Kathleen Sublette for her insightful editing.

To Darla Rockwood and Eugene Wheeler for the cover design.

To the members of the Ventura County Writer's Club nonfiction genre group, who supplied many excellent critiques along the way.

To Leonard Felder, Ph.D., best-selling author and therapist, who critiqued portions of the book and encouraged me to continue.

To James L. McGaugh, Ph.D., psychobiologist and former Dean of the School of Biological Sciences and Vice-Chancellor of the University of California at Irvine, who gave me valuable information on his research of the brain.

To Carl Cotman, Ph.D., Director of the Alzheimer's Disease Research Center on the Irvine campus, who provided me with pertinent facts about the latest Alzheimer's research.

To our relatives and friends, whose love and support sustained me.

Carol Heckman-Owen
Thousand Oaks, CA
December, 1991

PREFACE

A small voice has told me for some time to write about my husband Charlie and the lives we led since he developed Alzheimer's disease. I kept pushing the voice away. Why would I want to become involved with the difficult task of telling about this debilitating ailment, which has so drastically changed our lives?

Then I remembered all the research I had done to learn more about the illness; all the methods I used to care for Charlie; and all the soul-searching. I finally found hope for the future, thanks to the work around the world of dedicated scientists, who every day draw closer to a cure.

If this book can impart hope to others, who battle this disease in their families or their friends, my words may make it easier for them.

My book is about a most unusual romance, which began in high school, and was renewed after years of separation and the deaths of our spouses.

Some of the happiest days of my life followed our wedding. Then Charlie began to show dementia symptoms, which became worse as the months and years passed.

As our older population increases, spouses, children, grandchildren, and sometimes friends may be faced with these issues. May God be with you if you find yourself in a similar situation.

Carol Heckman-Owen

INTRODUCTION

Before you read about Charlie and me and the Alzheimer's disease that played havoc with our lives, perhaps it would help to read a few definitions to better understand the medical terms within the book. People often confuse dementia with the aging process.

What is dementia, and what is Alzheimer's Disease (AD)?

Dementia is the loss of intellectual functions such as thinking, remembering, and reasoning and sometimes changes in personality, mood, and behavior. Dementia is not a disease, and is not a normal part of the aging process. It is a group of symptoms. Dementia, or the loss of these functions, accompanies several diseases including Alzheimer's. In fact, the major causes of dementia are senile dementia of the Alzheimer's type and multi-infarct dementia.

Alzheimer's type, or SDAT (Senile Dementia, Alzheimer's Type) is a progressive degenerative disease characterized by gradual onset that attacks the brain and results in impaired memory, thinking, and behavior. It affects an estimated 2.5 million American adults. There is rapid loss of brain mass and the spread of "plaques" or neurofibrillary tangles throughout the brain. Ten to fifteen years usually elapse between the recognition of the disorder and the death of the patient.

Multi-Infarct Disorders, (MID), sometimes called vascular dementia, are the intellectual impairment syndromes related to strokes (infarcts) in the brain. The onset of MID may be relatively sudden as many strokes can occur before symptoms appear. These strokes may damage areas of the brain responsible for a specific function, such as calculations, and there may be more generalized symptoms, such as disorientation, confusion, and behavioral changes. As a result, MID may appear similar to Alzheimer's Disease. In fact, MID and Alzheimer's Disease co-exist in 15-20 percent of dementia patients.

Other diseases that are accompanied by dementia are:

Parkinson's Disease: A disorder of the nervous system characterized by rhythmic tremors and muscle rigidity, creating slowness of movement.

Amyotrophic Lateral Sclerosis (Lou Gehrig's Disease): A motor neuron disease characterized by progressive degeneration of the nervous system so that both voluntary and involuntary muscle control is lost.

Creutzfeldt-Jakob Disease (CJD): A rare fatal brain disease caused by a transmissible infectious agent, possibly a virus. Failing memory, changes in behavior, and a lack of coordination are some of the symptoms. It progresses rapidly, usually causing death within one year of diagnosis.

Huntington's Disease (HD): A hereditary disorder that usually begins in mid-life and is characterized by irregular involuntary movements of the limbs or facial muscles and intellectual decline. Psychiatric problems are common, with depression and memory disturbances occurring in early stages. (The pattern of memory disturbance is not the same as that seen in Alzheimer's patients).

Normal Pressure Hydrocephalus (NPH): An uncommon disorder that consists of difficulty in walking, dementia, and urinary incontinence. An obstruction in the normal flow of the spinal fluid causes the fluid to build up.

Pick's Disease: A rare brain disease which closely resembles Alzheimer's Disease and is usually difficult to clinically diagnose. Disturbances in personality, behavior, and orientation may precede and initially be more severe than memory defects. Like Alzheimer's Disease, a definitive diagnosis is usually obtained at autopsy.

Other conditions that are often confused with Alzheimer's are:

Senility: The lay term for dementia, a term which has fallen into disrepute because it implies irreversibility and has long been used for conditions that are reversible. Dementia is the more appropriate term because "senile" is defined as "relating to old age" and one need not be old to have dementia, and dementia is not a part of the normal aging process.

Depression: Often older people are diagnosed as having an irreversible brain condition, dementia, when the problem is depression. Depression is a psychiatric disorder marked by sadness, inactivity, difficulty in concentration, and feelings of hopelessness. Many severely depressed patients will have mental deficits including poor concentration and attention. When dementia and depression are present together, intellectual deterioration may be exaggerated. Depression, whether present alone or in combination with dementia, can be reversed with proper treatment.

Delirium: A collection of intellectual and behavioral deficits that are generally associated with treatable conditions. If identified quickly and treated, the patient usually returns to normal levels of intellectual ability. If not treated, many of the underlying diseases will produce a permanent dementia. Causes of delirium are reactions to medications or alcohol, malnutrition. and acute medical disorders including tumors, encephalitis, electrolytic imbalance, heart failure, and many others.

PART I

CHARLIE AND ME

One

THE STORY OF OUR ROMANCE

Many a man has fallen in love with a girl in a light
so dim he would not have chosen a suit by it.

Maurice Chevalier

In the late 1920s Charlie and I were high school sweethearts in Oak Park, a suburb of Chicago, Illinois. We met each other in August, shortly before the beginning of our junior year, through my friend, Mildred. (NOTE: Some names and places have been changed to protect the privacy of individuals.)

One evening her fiancé, Taylor, brought his buddy Charlie with him. A short time later, they walked across the street and joined me on our front porch.

The weather was hot and muggy - a typical summer night in our area. Before the days of air conditioning, most homes featured screened front porches, where families gathered on warm evenings, drank cold lemonade, and munched on cookies.

The moon was only a sliver that night. I didn't have a good look at Charlie nor he at me. He told me later that it was love *before* first sight. We talked and talked. As Charlie was leaving, he asked if I would play tennis with him the next day. Our tennis game led to more games and invitations to dances and theatres.

Charlie had a delightful sense of humor. We had many fun times together. I met his family and liked them. His father, Charles, Sr., beguiled us with outlandish stories. His mother, Vera, was an adorable, attractive blonde and a gourmet cook. His sister, Vaughn, and her boyfriend, who was also named Charlie, joined us on many of our dates.

My Charlie's parents loved to dance. Frequently they would take us to the other side of Chicago, where we floated across the floor to the tunes of the big bands. Charlie played the saxophone and piano and sang in our church choir. I admire anyone with a good voice as I can't even carry a tune.

In my sophomore year, I dated a boy named Howie. I broke up with him during the summer, but he wouldn't take "No" and kept pursuing me. After Charlie and I became a twosome, Charlie told him to back off, or he'd be sorry. One afternoon as I was walking out of school, Howie came over, put his arm through mine, and said he wanted me to be his girlfriend again. Charlie was waiting outside for me. When he saw that I was trying to pull away, he started a fight with Howie on the front lawn of the school grounds. Students flocked around, but no one interfered. I noticed Mr. Bennett, our vice-principal, standing in the doorway, but he made no move to break up the fight. Charlie was the victor and Howie never troubled me again.

Charlie's parents owned property in Wisconsin with a lake and two log cabins. During the next two years, all of the family spent many happy days up there, swimming, fishing, and hiking. The only bad part was Vera's insistence on making us eat huge onion sandwiches the first day to clean out our systems without anyone around to object to the odor. I detested onions and gritted my teeth before biting into one.

In high school, Charlie and I were in the same class, although he was three years older. I skipped fourth grade. A respiratory ailment prevented him from attending elementary school for more than a year.

We often studied together. He helped me with math, which I never liked, and I coached him in English and history.

There were three automobiles in Charlie's family — two Willys Knights and Charlie's Ford. His sister, four years older than Charlie, had first priority, so Charlie and I rode in his old Ford-no top, no windshield, and no fenders, with only a crank in front for a self starter and a box in back for a rumble seat. In winter I froze; in summer I roasted. When it rained or snowed, he threw a heavy canvas cover over me.

Both of us were active in our Methodist Church. He played on the basketball team. I taught a kindergarten class. On Sunday mornings, I played an old manual organ with my feet actively pumping the pedals for the youngsters to sing "Jesus Loves Me" and other children's hymns.

Church picnics were held on the banks of the Des Plaines River, where we enjoyed homemade delicacies of chicken, ham, potato salad, pies, and watermelon, engaged in competitive games, and canoed.

The parents of one of our Methodist Epworth League members owned a cabin at Long Lake, about forty miles from Oak Park. Several of our day outings for the entire membership were held there. I vividly recall one ride home in a blinding rain storm with lightning and thunder crashing around us and me huddled in fear under my canvas cover.

After most of the dances or movies, we drove out to a hot dog stand on the River Road, a favorite hangout for teenagers. My parents imposed a midnight curfew for me.

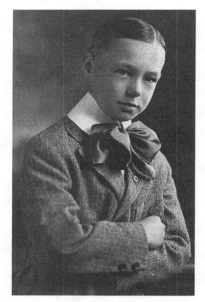

Charlie, Age 9

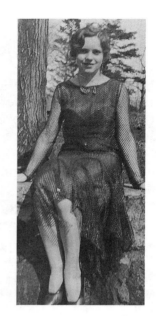

Carol, Age 17

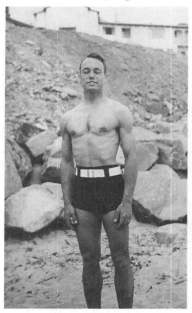

Charlie, life guard, 1926

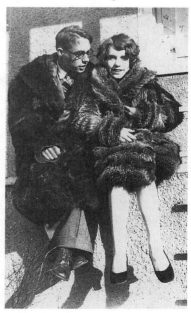

Charlie and Carol, 1928

Chapter One

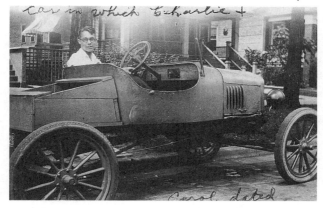

Car in which Charlie and Carol dated, 1927

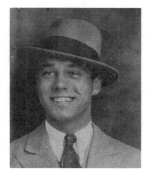

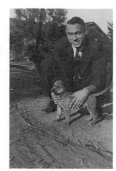

Charlie Owen, 1930   Charlie, 18, Oak Park, IL

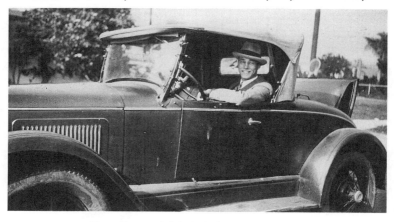

Charlie and his Whippet car, 1930

Many times we raced home at unsafe speeds to make the deadline. Years later, when our own children were out, I would say, "I want you home by midnight. If, for any reason, you see that you are not going to make it without speeding, phone and tell us why."

Like many teenagers in those days, our group had a particular Lovers' Lane in Thatcher's Woods about five miles from Oak Park. We often double dated with someone who had a closed car if we were unable to get one of Charlie's parents' cars. We talked, cuddled, and kissed. We even became friends with the police, who patrolled the grounds, looked into every car, and often stopped to chat with us.

Our junior and senior years were idyllic ones. Little did we know or worry about the future or what happiness, and then what despair, would engulf us. The word Alzheimer meant nothing to us nor to the majority of people in the 20s.

Ah, that Spring should vanish with the Rose!
That gentle sweetscented manuscript should close!

Edward Fitzgerald

Alas, most good happenings must come to an end. But life marches on.

Two

LOVE FOUND AND LOST

Take away love and our earth is a tomb.

Robert Browning

After graduation, I journeyed east to Wellesley College in Massachusetts: Charlie moved to California with his family. We continued writing until he alleges I sent him a "Dear John" letter and married Walter. Our correspondence dwindled to Christmas messages. Several years later Charlie joined the ranks of wedded bliss.

I fell in love with Walter in the summer before my freshman year in high school. We met at a party four blocks from where I lived. His athletic six-foot figure, dark wavy hair, and twinkling blue eyes captured my heart. After the party, he walked me home, stopping to give me a hug and kiss under the street light at each corner.

The next day, he and his bicycle appeared in our driveway. He said, "How about a game of tennis?" Off we went with me perched on the cross bar in front of him. On the way home, several of his buddies saw us and yelled, "Robbing the cradle!" He was a senior in high school. Our romance was over before it began, for he wouldn't look at me for another four years. In the meantime, I dated others, but finally settled on Charlie to be my steady boyfriend.

After college, I met Walter again and knew that he was the one for me. My correspondence with Charlie dwindled to exchanging Christmas cards. Before Walter asked me to marry him, he wanted to be assured that I loved children as much as he did. His best friend was married to a girl who refused to have any. I had already decided that I was never going to become pregnant. Babies meant diapers to be changed, spitting up, sleep disturbed, my freedom disrupted. I detested baby sitting. What did I want with all those horrible aspects of raising children? But, hypocrite that I was, I loved Walter and wanted to marry him. I pretended that I adored the little brats.

You can imagine how I felt when I learned several months after our marriage that I was pregnant. However, I soon became happy about my pregnancy.

Walter had just started a new business adventure - a telephone answering service for doctors. We were very poor. How could we afford a baby? Maybe all of us would starve. Maybe I would die in giving birth. My mother nearly lost her life when I was born. Then the thought that a new life had been entrusted to us took over, and I became a very happy mother-to-be with the enthusiastic support of an ecstatic father-to-be.

Nancy was a precious, blonde baby, who could always coo and gurgle at everything and everybody. She ate what the doctor ordered, slept the prescribed hours, and never kept us awake at night. I discovered that I loved being a mother. Our other two children were planned: Jay four years later; Susan seven years after Jay.

The business prospered. Life took on a rosy hue. Both of us worked many hours a week managing our telephone answering service, but those were happy years.

After eleven years of marriage, we decided to move to California, where my brother Ralph and his wife Ellen lived, and where my parents planned to retire the following year. We settled in San Marino. Walter became associated with a pharmaceutical company; I became a homemaker and volunteer in the community.

After forty years of married bliss, Walter died three hours after suffering a massive heart attack two days before Christmas as we were about to join friends and participate in the Newport Harbor Boat Parade of Lights. Depression overwhelmed me for several months. I poured out my sorrow in the following poem:

FOREVER LOVE

Sleep descends.
Moist eyed
I vow to greet
a fresh new dawn
again.

Death's stalking
figure strode through
my life
and captured
my heart,
my mate.

"Be strong! Be brave!"
All said to me.
The cadence of their words
marches off
the months and yet
I am alone.

Misery for my loved
and lost
still lingers,

Even as I reach
to touch the
promise of
the dawn.

My future seemed dark, but I had trust that the years ahead would be all right. Because Walter and I had saved, I had enough to live on and I felt that recovery would come by being close to my children, grandchildren, and by volunteering in worthwhile activities in the church and community.

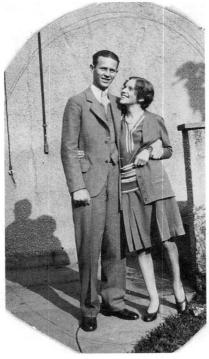

Carol,18, and Walter

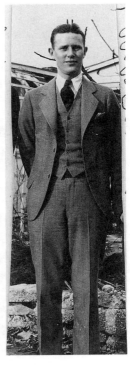

Walter, 21

Three

THE ONSET

Turn your scars into stars.
Robert Schuller

The following year Charlie and I were reunited while making plans with several members of our graduating class to return to Oak Park, Illinois, for a high school reunion.

He and I resumed our friendship as if there had been no time gap since school days. We felt like teenagers as we held hands and walked along winding paths in California's Fountain Valley park, fragrant with flowering trees and shrubs. Charlie had retired from the postal service after 31 years; I joined the University of California at Irvine in 1965, eight months before it opened to students, and retired after nine years of many challenges as assistant to the Dean of Biological Sciences.

Our friendship blossomed into love. In September of 1977, we exchanged marriage vows in the gardens of the University of California at Irvine. At the ceremony, Charlie, sixty-eight years young, stood five feet, eight inches tall and wore a natural Yul Brunner haircut. He was my knight in shining armor. His blue suit matched the blue of his eyes. I wore a white lace over sea-green taffeta gown. A wreath of miniature yellow roses encircled my brown hair, tinged with a few flecks of grey. The top of my head reached up to Charlie's nose. As we gazed at each other, his eyes seemed to penetrate into my soul. I felt reborn and knew that joy could once again be mine.

Marriage brought other blessings. I now had the large caring family I always wanted, the offspring of his previous two marriages.

Another joy was resumption of marital relations. Yes, I do enjoy sex. Masters and Johnson wrote, "If you have sex twice a week while you are 40, when you are 90, you will do the same, barring significant illness or the death of a mate." In our case, a new dimension of spiritual love and closeness entered the picture to give it still more meaning.

The next few years were some of the happiest in my life. I found it enchanting to awaken each morning and hear, "You are the most beautiful girl in the whole wide world, and I love you more than words can say."

Charlie and I decided not to live in his home in the San Gabriel area or mine in Orange County. We wanted to make an entirely new life for ourselves and chose Camarillo Springs, thirty-five miles north of Los Angeles and seven miles from the ocean. In our new location, we took long walks, swam, played golf, participated in volunteer activities, and found some wonderful new friends.

Before I married Charlie, I made plans to visit the Orient with our former minister, Thatcher Jordan, his wife Vivian, and several friends. I told Charlie, "I'm not twenty-two any longer, and I want to make this trip. I hope you will go with me, but if you won't, I intend to go. Will you wait for me? Do you still want to marry me?" The answer was a resounding "Yes."

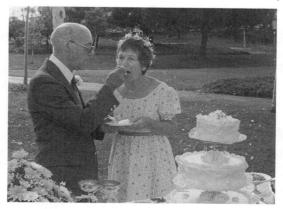

Wedding Day for Carol and Charlie

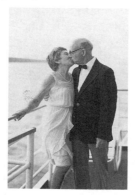

Carol and Charlie on their Honeymoon Cruise

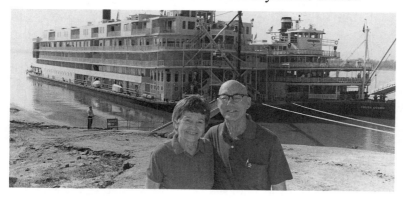

Carol and Charlie in front of the Mississippi Queen

Charlie had never flown in a plane. His former wife was afraid to fly because a plane crash had made her a widow. Several friends suggested that Charlie and I fly on a short trip to San Francisco first. "No way," I responded, "I had several scary experiences on that flight when the planes left San Francisco on beautiful sunny afternoons only to run into fog. We would land in Ontario and be bused to our Orange County airport. If we take off from Los Angeles International, our first stop will be Honolulu, and Charlie can't disembark until then."

Charlie not only joined me but truly enjoyed the trip. The plane took off and landed twenty-six times while visiting Japan, Taiwan, Bangkok, Singapore, and the Philippines. He was as calm as if he had flown all his life and was not even disturbed when we were diverted from Singapore to Kuala Lumpur because of an accident on Singapore's runway. Several weeks later we sat for six hours on Japan's bullet train when it stalled because of tangled wires overhead. Charlie took all of this in stride. At that time, there were no obvious signs that he was suffering from Alzheimer's disease.

In retrospect, I believe that this malady began to take hold even before we were married. On our honeymoon, we drove from California to Missouri, where Charlie's son Rod and his family lived, and then on to Oak Park for our high school reunion. On the way, we sang the good old songs of that era when Ray Noble, Benny Goodman, the Dorsey Brothers, and other big bands charmed the populace. We exchanged reminiscences from our dating days. I am blessed with an excellent memory, but Charlie's recollections of those years were better than mine. Later I learned that Alzheimer patients remember childhood and teenage events better than recent happenings.

An incident, which I thought amusing then, came back to haunt me later. We stopped to buy milk, crackers, and cheese for picnic lunches along the way. The parking lot at the market was crowded. I asked Charlie to let me out in front of the store. He refused. He had been overly-protective of me, so I testily said, "What do you think could possibly happen if I went in alone?" He laughingly replied, "The butcher might grind you up for hamburgers." Charlie's fear of being by himself or getting lost is a symptom of Alzheimer's, which was not apparent to me at the time.

As the days marched on, I realized that he needed me for a safety blanket. He wanted to be with me constantly. Since we were still newlyweds, I did not mind at first. Then I felt smothered.

Thanksgiving arrived shortly after our trip back east. We celebrated with Charlie's stepchildren in San Jose, California. For dessert, I was asked if I wanted Charlie's choice. "What's that?" I inquired. Marge, his stepdaughter, replied, "Barbara always makes three pies for holidays: apple, mince, and pumpkin. Charlie can never make up his mind which he wants, so we always give him a slice of each one." Inability to make decisions is another symptom of the disease.

As the necessity of making other choices arose, I found myself making more and more of them. "Where shall we go for dinner?" "What would you like to watch on television?" "Should we go to see 'Oklahoma' at the Moorpark Theatre?" Charlie always answered, "Whatever you want to do." At first, his consideration pleased me. Later, it became a source of irritation until I realized that he couldn't help himself. Like the actress in "The Flower Drum Song," I enjoy being a girl and am happy to have a man take care of me, but Charlie and I were now reversing our roles.

By 1981, Charlie's strange behavior and conversation patterns became a source of worry. No longer could he remember simple facts or even the names of some of his closest friends. He misplaced belongings frequently and felt that someone was entering our home and stealing them. One day I found his shaver in the refrigerator and his best pair of slacks in the trash.

Disorientation became a way of life. Disorientation is a cold, objective, clinical word that conveys nothing of the human feelings of fear and panic which Charlie must have been experiencing when he became conscious of not knowing where he was or what was happening to his mind and body.

I first realized that Charlie was losing his memory when I said to him, "Charlie, will you please take these cans out to the trash and bring back the bottle of turpentine?" He took care of the cans but couldn't remember what else I had asked him to do. About the same time I became constantly aware of what he was saying to others, as his conversation often didn't make any sense. Gradually, pangs of anxiety—not sharp at first, but, nevertheless, painful, came over me. At this point, I knew some professional help was needed.

In October of 1981, we sat with fear and trepidation in the office of our family physician, Dr. Bonin. He gave Charlie a thorough physical examination and administered some simple psychological tests. The following is part of their conversation:

Doctor: "Who is President of our United States?"

Charlie: "I can't remember his name, but he was an actor in California."

Doctor: "His name is Reagan. Who was President before Reagan?"

Charlie: "I don't know his name either, but he makes peanut butter."

Dr. Bonin and I chuckled. Even Charlie joined in our outburst of laughter despite his not knowing why.

The doctor informed us that he was referring Charlie to a neurologist and a psychologist for further tests. He instructed me to ask Charlie questions every day and to repeat them frequently without fail.

Several days later I asked Charlie, "Who is President of our United States?" He immediately answered, "Reagan, of course. Everyone knows that. Why are you asking me such a dumb question?" He had no recollection of his visit to Dr. Bonin. Most dementia patients alternate between lucidity and incoherence.

I wondered what would happen next. What would the referral doctors tell us? Hopefully, the problem might be a minor one, which diet and medication could solve. During this time, my children and friends were a source of comfort to me with their acceptance of Charlie and their understanding and support of me.

The psychologist, Dr. Mary Forner, was a charming, pleasingly-plump woman with beautiful grey hair and twinkling blue eyes. She appeared to be a caring person. Her motherly demeanor put Charlie at his ease, but her tests elicited no new information.

The neurologist, Dr. George Logan, was a tall, handsome rugged individual with piercing brown eyes. He wore a huge black bow tie and pointed cowboy boots, which fascinated Charlie. Following several tests, Dr. Logan said, "I want Charlie to have a CAT scan to be certain a tumor on the brain is not causing the problem. However, I feel positive that he has Alzheimer's. He shows all of the symptoms. Unfortunately, we doctors do not know what causes it or how to cure it."

I felt as though a rug had been pulled out from under me and I was falling into a deep, dark pit. Tension built up in my body. My stomach churned. How could I handle the situation? I went into a daze for the next few weeks.

Dr. Logan explained that Alzheimer's Disease is a disorder, characterized by degeneration of certain parts of the brain producing intellectual impairment. The condition was first identified by a German neurologist, Alois Alzheimer, in 1906. His words struck a death knell in my body. I tried to pull myself together but only partially succeeded. My hopes centered on all the research programs and advances in the medical field. Surely Charlie could be helped.

My attention returned to the surroundings in Dr. Logan's office as he elaborated on the disease and read the following:

> *"Alzheimer's begins with memory loss. An individual may forget the date and possibly his address. Then it really sneaks up on him. After awhile, he cannot remember where he puts objects. He may even get lost. He becomes irritable and agitated, but refuses to believe that anything is wrong. The condition becomes worse. Alzheimer's is a progressive disease with no known cure at this time. Do not confuse it with senility, which is a symptom of a specific disease. Some conditions similar to Alzheimer's are treatable; others like Alzheimer's are not. After a thorough checkup that will exclude other ailments causing memory loss, we doctors assume that the patient has Alzheimer's. Only an autopsy will confirm diagnosis."*

Dr. Logan went on to say that changes in nerve cells and nerve ends disrupt nerve transmission between brain cells and cause the brain to malfunction.

The room started spinning before my eyes. My heart pounded furiously. I felt as though my whole world was falling apart and that I was in a long dark tunnel from which there was no escape. Alzheimer's happened only to others. No way could my Charlie be affected — he, who wrote beautiful music, played the piano and saxophone, enjoyed golf and tennis, practiced jujitsu, karate, and tai chi, delivered Meals On Wheels to shut-ins, and participated in many church and community affairs. At our monthly church dinners for the Circuit Riders' group, he received the official title of "Jokester" for the humorous stories with which he entertained the audience.

In 1981, few people were familiar with this dreaded disease. I knew about it through a stricken neighbor, Dean Triggs, former superintendent of the Ventura County school system. He continued to have a delightful sense of humor long after the disease struck. On one of his wife's visits to the hospital, where she finally had to place him, Betsy found him, wheelchair bound, in a section off limits to patients.

Betsy: "Dean, what are you doing out here?"

Dean: "Chasing the girls, what else?"

My attention returned to Dr. Logan as he went on to say that Alzheimer's strikes all levels of society and can begin as early as forty years of age. Further tests during the next couple of weeks confirmed Dr. Logan's finding.

A week after our visit with the doctor, CBS showed a documentary, stating that fifteen percent of individuals over sixty-five have Alzheimer's. I began to feel humiliated, helpless, and angry. I realized I was not yet ready to accept my husband's illness. Charlie denied that anything was wrong, but I could sense his own frustrations.

The seriousness of our situation had not fully penetrated. Then the ramifications sank in. I knew I had to face reality. But how? It was one of the most traumatic experiences of my life. I could not ignore the future and the way our lives would change. I would have to steel myself to cope.

I have a Pollyannaish attitude toward life and a tendency to bury my head in the sand like an ostrich when unpleasantness surrounds me. However, I do try to follow what I believe is my philosophy of life: an enduring trust in a power greater than ours, the Golden Rule, my Wellesley College's motto, "Non ministrari, sed ministrar" (Not to be ministered unto, but to minister).

A motto on my bedroom wall reads:

I

Have

Peace

There is nothing that can happen to me

that God and I cannot handle

- Together -

Now, how do I live up to the above? If Betsy Triggs could be a loving, caring person and cope with her husband's illness, surely I could do no less. I pulled myself together and decided that a beginning might be trying to learn patience, of which I have little, find some humor in Charlie's behavior no matter how disturbing it might be, and pray.

I remembered watching television one Sunday morning when the flu bug laid me low and I could not attend my own church. Dr. Robert Schuller of the Crystal Cathedral in Garden Grove, California, gave the sermon. His message came over loud and clear. "Turn your scars into stars." I realized that without God's abiding love, we are powerless. Our problems are too much to bear on our own. When we give them over to the Lord, we find strength and courage to carry on.

Since I believe that God helps those who help themselves, I began working on patience and how to cultivate it.

Four

PRAYER, PATIENCE and LAUGHTER

Life does not cease to be funny when people die, any more than it ceases to be serious when people laugh.

George Bernard Shaw

Not that I was always patient. Sometimes I would rush into our bedroom, hold the pillow over my mouth, and scream. Other times I would pound it until I thought the cover would rip and spread the down stuffing all over the room.

But I tried to remember that dementia patients are not deliberately stubborn, mean, or suspicious. Their behavior is beyond rational explanation. I attempted to keep our home as serene as possible. I permitted Charlie to help me as one would let a small child assist in baking cookies or setting the table even though it meant more effort and time on my part. No longer did I ask him to do more than one task at a time as one was all his memory could hold. If he acted in an irrational manner, I tried to distract him.

Again, I stressed laughing with him at every opportunity. Laughter is good for one's health. Doctors and hos-

27

pitals are beginning to discover the positive healing powers of laughter. In 1987, a publication of the American Association of Retired Persons stated that patients at DeKalb General Hospital in Decatur, Georgia, receive an unusual prescription — a few hours in a humor room. Instead of any medical equipment, they view videotapes of old movies in which Laurel and Hardy, W.C. Fields, and other comics are featured. Many who have lost interest in life revive and want to get well. Humor rooms have been discovered in other cities: Orlando, Florida; Schenectady, New York; Houston, Texas; Phoenix, Arizona; and Los Angeles, California. Somehow laughter enervates the endorphin glands to promote healing.

I felt that humor would benefit both of us. I began to monitor our television programs toward comical shows. "Laugh and the world laughs with you. Cry and you cry alone," is a saying I have heard for years. Therefore, I made up my mind that I would not complain about our situation to anyone.

And, most important, I talked with God about my problems and asked for his help. I tried not to pity myself for I remembered the story about the man who complained because he had no shoes until he met a man who had no feet.

Some days were good; some bad as Charlie seemed to improve, remained the same, or worsened. In February of 1982, Andrew Bonin, our family doctor, discontinued prescribing Halazone for memory loss since Charlie showed no improvement in that area. During the next year, Charlie seemed to be on a plateau.

In April of 1983, I learned about an Alzheimer support group, meeting in Ventura, a neighboring city, the following day. I wondered if attending would help or hurt Charlie, but decided to go. During the time we were there, he didn't seem disturbed despite the fact that the film "Someone I Used to Know" was depressing. He sat quietly at my side, but I felt he had not understood anything being shown or said by the psychiatrist and nurse, who were present to answer caregivers' questions.

I found it comforting to be with others, who were sharing the same problems. Before our departure, I bought the caregivers' "Bible," *The 36-hour Day.* While the book was helpful, I could not follow some of its suggestions. One about placing locks on all doors and windows was out of the question. I knew Charlie well enough that if I carried out this advice, he would smash the glass to get out, as he was beginning to wander, another symptom of Alzheimer's.

Many victims of this disease function fairly well during the day, but after sundown they become restless, confused, and have difficulty sleeping, say experts. These patients suffer from a strange syndrome called "sundowning." Doctors aren't sure of the cause. Dr. Howard Crystal, assistant professor of neurology at Albert Einstein College of Medicine, wrote, "Alzheimer's gradually destroys the mind. A victim who suffers from sundowning may awaken in darkness and not know where he is. He may panic. Or, he might awaken and have to go to the bathroom, but not remember where it is. In his confusion, he may wander out of the house while searching for it." Here are some tips on how sundowning victims can be helped.

- Install a night light.
- Provide a bedside commode. This may be less upsetting.
- Install an alarm system to alert you if the patient strays outside.
- Use "child-safe" doorknob covers. They fit loosely over the doorknob so only the cover - not the knob itself turns.
- Fence your yard.

- Use brighter lights.
- Discourage excessive napping during the day.

I tried to stay awake at night in order to hear Charlie leaving his bed but found it impossible.

About two o'clock one morning, I saw a large man standing in our bedroom doorway. I froze until he said, "Don't be frightened, Carol. It's only Marv." Marv and Marge were close neighbors and good friends. He went on to say, "Charlie is over at our house in a very disoriented condition. He told us you locked him out, but the front door was wide open when I came over." The next morning Charlie remembered nothing about the previous evening's events.

Wanderings both day and night increased. I did not worry too much during the day as we lived in a gated community, where all of my neighbors knew him and would bring him back home. But one evening at dusk while we were staying with my son Jay and daughter-in-law Darla in Orange County, he slipped out of the house without our seeing him. When we realized that he was missing, we walked and drove around all nearby streets. No sign of him. About eleven p.m., we phoned the police. Nothing. At four in the morning, the phone rang. Betty Adair, one of our good friends in Fountain Valley, said that Charlie was there with swollen, sore feet, utterly exhausted and disoriented. She and her husband Norm were putting him to bed. We immediately drove approximately eight miles to their home. Charlie was asleep. When he awakened, he had no memory of where he had been or why he had left us.

Other incidents followed.

Five

PROGRESSION OF DISEASE

Life is like an onion. You peel it off one layer at a time, and sometimes you weep.

Carl Sandberg

One night I saw Charlie standing in the middle of our bedroom. "What do you want," I asked. He responded, "I don't know what to do or where to go." I led him back to bed. Other times we talked. Eventually he would return to bed or go out and lie on the davenport. We finally gave up our queen size bed and bought two twin beds, as Charlie bounced up and down in a way that my rest was gradually getting less and less. We put the twin beds next to each other, which partially satisfied him. An oversized comforter appeared to have only one bed underneath it.

One day Charlie misplaced his keys. I knew he had them a couple of hours previously as he opened the door when we returned from a shopping expedition. He could not comprehend that the keys must be some place at home since we had not left the house since then. He wanted me to call friends, where we had dined the previous evening, and our daughter in Bell Canyon. I finally found the keys tucked under a sofa pillow.

Charlie's memory for numbers or calculations was fading. At the time of our marriage, he and I decided that I would give him enough money at the beginning of each month to cover half of the household expenses, and he would pay all of the bills.

In the summer of 1983, he received a letter from the bank informing him that his account was overdrawn. He showed it to me and asked, "What should I do about this?" I did not see how his finances could be in the red, as I had a pretty fair idea of what our income and expenses were. I asked to see his checkbook. To my astonishment and dismay, I found that he had been sending $5.00 checks to every organization requesting donations. He sheepishly said, "They asked me for it." Also, he had not balanced his checkbook for six months. After all his years of keeping meticulous accounts, he had now forgotten how to. At this point, I took charge of the family finances.

As far as his personal needs were concerned, I told him when to bathe and frequently had to turn the knobs. He had been accustomed to taking a shower every morning. Now he would say, "I just had one." I did not insist. He wasn't going to die because he didn't bathe every day. One morning after I turned on the water and told him to get in the shower, as several days had elapsed since his last one, he retorted "I've already had four today. Are you going to make me take another one?" Brushing his teeth became a major chore, bitterly protested by Charlie despite my concern not to hurt him. Most days necessity forced me to shave him.

I began to see why Alzheimer patients often turn on their loved ones, for I felt Charlie was beginning to perceive me as his jailer.

Later, I said, "Charlie, your granddaughter Rose with her husband Bob and their three children will be coming from Oklahoma to visit us next week." Charlie responded, "Who is she? Why are they coming?" The previous day he had asked how they were and wondered why they never came to see us.

About this time Charlie reached a point of arguing about his clothes. For almost seven years of our marriage, we had never had an argument - unbelievable, but true.

In 1983, paranoia joined his inability to make decisions and to care for himself. One morning he insisted that a pair of slacks he had worn the previous day would kill him if worn again. He would not go ten feet away from the house without locking the doors. He insisted that someone was lurking around the corner of our home to "case the joint."

Charlie thought that Tony, one of our neighbors, was out to get him. On our morning walk, he made us detour around Paseo Margarita to avoid seeing Tony. That night he took the bucket of wood, which sat next to the fireplace, out to the porch. He said it was making him sick.

From our kitchen window, I could watch him in the driveway as he performed his weekly chore of placing plastic trash bags near the curb for pick-up. I could hardly believe my eyes when I saw him turn one bag upside down and shake the contents on the ground. He came rushing into the house, exclaiming, "Some man dumped trash all over our yard. Go out and get him." The repetition of this statement all during the day set my nerves on edge. Several times I took him out in the car while we drove around looking for this strange individual. I wondered how much longer situations similar to the above could go on without losing my mind.

Not all days were bad. Some of the good times included picnics on the beach, dinner dances, and visits with friends.

Elderhostel programs from 1982 to 1984 provided many of the good days. What is Elderhostel? It is a melange of exciting adventures to make life richer and more meaningful. Elderhostels are held all over the world year-round, usually on college campuses, with some in such exotic places as Egypt, India, and China. Participants sixty years or over, or fifty for an accompanying companion, receive a smorgasbord of activities.

I learned about Elderhosteling from my attorney son, Jay. He phoned one evening with a great deal of excitement in his voice and said, "Mom, I have just heard about a program I know you will love." He and his spouse Darla had dined with a client and his wife that evening and found them enthusiastic about Elderhosteling in Australia. I wrote for their brochure and settled on Brigham Young's offerings at Provo, Utah, since the University was on the way to an already-planned visit with Charlie's granddaughter Connie, her husband Bob, and their baby son in Vail, Colorado.

One of the three subjects offered Monday through Friday mornings was "Learning and Memory," which I thought might help our situation. Sorry to say it didn't. But the classes, with no exams or participation unless one desired, supplemented by field trips, proved ideal for our situation. At that time, Charlie's memory caused problems, but not enough to disturb other people.

Other Elderhostel trips to Anchorage, Alaska, and Hidden Valley, California, followed. I realized while we were in Hidden Valley that this would be our last Elderhostel trip together. The men in the group were wonderful about helping Charlie shower and taking him into the bathroom, but I felt that I was imposing.

On one of our trips we visited New Orleans, where we boarded the Mississippi Queen for a week's cruise up to Vicksburg. From the time we left until we returned, Charlie was so afraid he would be lost that he stuck to me like glue. Our stateroom had a bath, so I managed to take care of him, with difficulty. I have to admit that my patience was sorely tried. I became exasperated many times and then was ashamed of myself, as I knew he couldn't help his actions, which ranged from interrupting when I tried to talk with some of the passengers, eating more than anybody else, and trying to leave our stateroom while he was naked.

One evening during the cruise when we were in the middle of the Mississippi River, the steward began pouring wine in my glass during dinner. Charlie immediately shouted, "Don't give her any wine. She has to drive." The steward was superb. He responded, "It's perfectly all right for her to have it. I always collect all of the car keys before dinner." Our four delightful dinner companions were highly amused and burst into gales of laughter along with people at the surrounding tables, who had witnessed the scene.

In December of 1983, Charlie began writing our return address on Christmas envelopes. He finished several, then turned to me and said he did not know how to write any more. I tried to show him, but he couldn't form the letters. However, an hour later he handed me the following almost-unintelligible note:

"Dear Honie!

I'm sorry, but I can't help due to the stuff I get. I'm trying, but can't due much.

I love you!"

Charlie's command of grammar and spelling had been excellent. I envied his penmanship with its beautiful swirling curves. The tears rolled down my cheeks. I cried for both of us. My heart ached for his torment, evident from the expression on his face and from his shaking body.

About this time Charlie's operation of our automobile alarmed me. I tried to take over to no avail. He made lane changes on the freeway but did not signal until we had already entered the new lane. When I remonstrated, he said, "I did too signal." One morning he sat in our car on the driveway but did not turn on the ignition. Then he frightened me by grabbing the gear shift, shaking it so hard

I thought it would break, and saying, "What do I do with this?"

I telephoned Dr. Logan, Charlie's neurologist, who promised to handle the situation and gave us an appointment for the next day. I told Charlie it was time for his check-up, and the doctor wanted me to drive so that he could rest on the way down. At the doctor's office, Charlie was given an ultimatum he did not want to accept but was forced to.

I had driven no more than a dozen times during our marriage. Charlie took me everywhere and waited in the car even though some of my luncheons or meetings might last for several hours. Finally, I gave up going any place without him, as I could no longer leave him alone in the car.

From our home in Camarillo Springs, entry onto the highway driving south came midpoint on a steep incline, with trucks thundering behind us as they picked up speed to make the hill. Charlie made me nervous. He sat on the edge of his seat, giving me directions, which I could not execute without endangering our lives as well as others. He would tell me to get in the other lane. If I had followed his instructions, there would have been one grand pile-up of cars and people. Then he would say, "Damn it! You never do what I tell you." I feared he might grab the wheel. Thank the Lord, he never did, but my stomach felt as though it was tied in knots many times.

Housekeeping involved dusting by me and vacuuming by Charlie until he couldn't remember where he had cleaned. I tried to direct him by saying, "Go in the back bedroom next." He angrily replied, "I've already been there. Do you want me to do it again?" From a friend I learned about two young ladies, who operated their own cleaning service, bringing all of the necessary equipment with them. They were jewels and my bridge over troubled waters.

In 1984, I heard about a research program on problems of the aging, funded by a government grant to the University of California at Los Angeles and the Veterans' Administration. After several interviews and examinations, Charlie was accepted. Placebos were given to half of the group; the rest received Trental, a medication which European doctors found successful with many Alzheimer patients' symptoms, but which had not as yet been approved in the United States.

In the beginning, we drove the seventy-mile round trip three times a week for a two-to-three hour session, then once a week, and finally once a month during a six-month period. One day Charlie told the psychologist that his ears were stopped up and he couldn't breathe through them.

Friends and family told me how much better Charlie seemed. We learned later that he had been on the placebo. I wondered whether it was all the attention he received from psychologists, psychiatrists, technicians, and other personnel that made the difference.

Trental was one of the many medications thought to cure or curb Alzheimer's. Since then I have scoured medical reports to keep abreast of ongoing research, but no cure has appeared.

During that period, I saw Charlie one morning in our driveway holding an oil can and looking at the battery in our car. I asked him what he intended oiling, to which he replied, "The batteries are low. I need to fill them." Only the utmost persuasion on my part succeeded in making him put away the can and permit me to take the car to a local garage.

As mentioned before, some days were better than others. He babbled many times, but usually would say something after remarks of mine even though his words were not relevant. Our good friend, Joe Keller, remarked that Charlie always had an answer for everything but not always the solution.

We still participated in a weekly cribbage group. Since he could no longer remember how to play the game, both of us would become one. I would ask him, "Is this the right card to play?" He always responded in the affirmative. While his speech had become incoherent most of the time, our families and friends were patient with him, even listening when he babbled.

Charlie received the official title of jokester for our Circuit Riders' group at the church and told a joke every month for several years at their dinners. He had not been able to for some time until one night early in the spring of 1985, a friend handed him a joke. I asked Elva, our president, if he should try to give it. Irene Roberts, standing nearby, said, "Let him do it. We all love him so much that even if he flubs it, we'll all clap." Charlie gave it with no problems.

It wasn't the apple in the Garden of Eden that caused all the trouble. It was the pear (pair) on the ground. (M.D.O'Connor)

Applause was overwhelming. Afterward, a number of our members came over to tell him how happy they were to have him tell a joke again.

During 1985, Charlie's memory seemed worse, but his conversation became clearer. One day he asked me to make a 'W.' I showed him how. He put one 'W' on the paper and then continued to make 'W's' all down the page. On the way to our daughter's that night, he asked me about thirty times where we were going and why. My innards churned.

In March of that year, Charlie collapsed during the sermon and fell over the church pew in front of us. Our minister asked if there was a doctor or nurse in the congregation. A doctor, nurse, and therapist came over. An usher wheeled in oxygen. Paramedics rushed him to the nearest hospital, Pleasant Valley in Camarillo. Then Kaiser's ambulance arrived and moved him to Humana

West Hills Hospital in Canoga Park, where Kaiser rented space while their own hospital was being built in Woodland Hills.

The doctor there said that all tests were negative, but they would keep him overnight for observation. While I was dressing the next morning, Charlie phoned, "Where are you? I want to go home. Why aren't you here?" He sounded frightened to be there without me.

In April of 1985, came more excitement. Paramedics arrived in the middle of the night to transport me to the emergency room at Pleasant Valley Hospital. After an examination and X-rays, the heart specialist phoned Kaiser to say that I was in no condition to be moved. I remained there for two days in the intensive care unit. Final diagnosis — angina and gallstones.

Two months later I suffered another night attack with the same hospital stay and same diagnosis. My daughter Susan and her husband Arlen took care of Charlie during my illnesses.

A few days after I returned, I saw Charlie trying unsuccessfully to hammer a stake into the ground. Ted, our next-door neighbor, saw him laboring and came over with a friend to finish the job. Later Charlie said, "I never want to see them again. They want to kill me."

That night I found Charlie standing in the middle of the bedroom, not knowing how to get ready for bed. He said, "What should I do with my shoes — take them off or leave them on tonight?"

One day in our car with the air conditioner operating, Charlie said he needed more air. I told him to roll down the window. He opened the door. Fortunately, we had just entered the freeway onramp and I stopped. Since Charlie refused to use a seatbelt, he probably would have flown out if we had gone a few more feet.

I awakened one night to find him standing in the middle of our bedroom sobbing. I went over, hugged him, and asked, "What's the trouble, Darling?" to which he pathetically replied, "I'm so sorry. I don't know. I really don't know." My poor dear! What was going to happen to him and to me? I had reached a point where I felt almost as confused as he was. Where would I find more ways to help us? I thought I could cope, but I began to wonder. He was in the second of the four stages of Alzheimer's. He was losing speech and misunderstanding what he heard. No longer could he follow a story line. What will I do as he reaches the other stages? (These phases or stages are discussed in detail in Chapter Eight).

Already my sleep was broken — I, who used to sleep like a log. He was up and down numerous times during the night. Try as hard as I could to keep control, I found that I was becoming nervous and jumpy. I became a compulsive eater, particularly of sweets with chocolate given a high priority.

By August of 1986, I had to bathe, shave, and dress him almost every day. Then on the first day of September, he took a shower without being told and dressed himself. That afternoon we played ping pong. Did he really have Alzheimer's? Dare I hope?

I did know that I needed more help. Through the Senior Citizen organization in our city, I learned about a day-care center. The fee was nominal, and Charlie was admitted for one day a week. What a glorious relief to have six hours free! I read without any interruptions, lunched with friends, and rested. Charlie resisted going at first but finally accepted his new situation with calmness and enjoyed the activities and the people.

As a stipulation of Charlie being in the day-care center, I was required to attend a number of meetings and lectures. One, given by Dr. Lanyard Dial, Director of Geriatric Services for Ventura County Health Care Agency, focused on the four stages of Alzheimer's. I realized that while I thought Charlie was in the second stage, he was also showing some symptoms of the other phases.

Six

FINAL DECISION

Put God to work for you and maximize your potential in our divinely ordered system.

Norman Vincent Peale

Only patience, humor, and prayer kept me from going berserk. Several months of as much serenity as one can expect with an Alzheimer patient provided the calm before the storm.

Charlie experienced no problems with continence during the day with the exception of slight dribblings in his shorts. At night he knew enough to find the bathroom but not enough to urinate or defecate into the toilet. I asked him many times to awaken me, but he never remembered. He refused to use diapers. No way could I stay awake all night. Finally, I placed old towels over the bathroom floor and cleaned up the mess each morning. He could not understand that Alzheimer's was the culprit. I told him that he was not to blame and tried my utmost to preserve his dignity. He kept saying, "I wouldn't do such a nasty thing. Go out and find the one who broke into our house and did this." That same remark was repeated over and over again all through the day. I wanted to scream.

Many frustrations occur, not because of major faults but from little aggravations day after day. So it was in my case - the constant repetitions, the incoherent speech, and the fear that something disastrous would happen to him. The final straw occurred early one morning in November of 1986. I have always had a weak stomach. I cleaned up the bathroom mess with my body shaking and tears pouring down my cheeks. How much more can I take?

Now comes the eerie part. My daughter Susan phoned that day. She knew from my voice that something was wrong. When I informed her of the problem, about which I had never told anyone previously, she said, "Mother I dreamt that Charlie tried to drink apple juice from the corner of his mouth and spilled it on the carpet. When I attempted to take away the glass, he resisted by hitting me." She went on to say that the alarm clock interrupted her dream at six-thirty, which was the exact time I cleaned the bathroom down on my hands and knees with utter hopelessness.

Later that day, I confided in Sally, a close friend. "Carol," she said, "God was telling your daughter that you needed help."

For over six months, my children and many of our friends and neighbors had urged me to put Charlie in a care home. Susan said, "Mother, you know I care about Charlie. He is the nicest, kindest man I have ever known, but I can see what he is doing to you, and I want you to live a lot longer."

The thought of parting with Charlie horrified me. I would never stoop to "putting him away." While the day care center gave me some respite, I realized I needed more. I tried to bring someone into our home. Charlie became infuriated. "What are you trying to do, get a baby sitter for me?" As the months passed, I knew I could no longer care for him. I had said many times that I would never place Charlie in a care home. But the time finally came, after urging by my family and friends, when I realized that this was the only solution to our problems.

One of my friends gave me "The Caregiver Bill of Rights," source unknown.

CAREGIVER'S BILL OF RIGHTS

- The right to live out our own life and retain our dignity and sense of self.
- The right to choose a plan of caring that accommodates our needs and the needs of those we care about.
- The right to be recognized as a vital and stabilizing source within our families.
- The right to be free of guilt, anguish, and doubt knowing that the decisions we make are appropriate for our own well-being and that of our loved one.
- The right to be ourselves enough to have confidence that we are doing the best we are able.

I read these and realized if I refused to change our life style, I would not be of any use to either Charlie or myself. By considering these caregiver rights, the disabled and frail elderly will be provided the highest and best care that we are capable of giving, and we may take pride in ourselves. After much thought and many prayers, everything began to fall into place like clockwork.

I remembered hearing about Rosewood through neighbors, whose daughter Cheryl and husband owned a residential care facility. I phoned her for an appointment to have Charlie, Susan, and me meet with her and Gwen, the administrator.

When we entered Rosewood, the friendly ambience gave us a comforting feeling. The staff seemed caring and competent. A bed in a pleasant double room with lush greenery outside the window was available. The $850.00 a month seemed reasonable. Rosewood is between a retirement facility and a nursing home, which met Charlie's needs at that time. After a thorough physical and mental examination, Rosewood accepted him. He entered three days later.

I explained to Charlie that I needed a good long rest. He seemed content to stay for my sake. Rosewood did not want me to visit him for several days in order for the staff to orient him to his new environment. On my first visit, Charlie said, "Are you rested enough? Can you take me home now?" His unhappiness clearly showed when I said I needed more time.

I knew I had made the right decision, but guilt feelings overwhelmed me. Articles I read about keeping aging parents or spouses at home until death added to my misery. One in the March 27, 1988 issue of "Los Angeles Times Magazine" by Gerald W. Haslam was particularly upsetting even though I read it months later. He told of the family confronting his father's progressive debilitation with compassion and patience. Mr. Haslam's mother lived in a nearby mobile home park, but was unable to take care of her husband. The family had help five days a week, so his and his wife's work schedules were little altered. Their children adjusted to being dislodged from their rooms and learned valuable lessons while caring for their grandfather. From Mr. Haslam's description of his father's ailments, he in no way had reached a stage where it might be necessary to place him in a care home.

After reading this beautiful tribute to an entire family, I experienced more guilt feelings, but logic finally rescued me. My case of being a lone caregiver was different. I realized that no one person in the Haslam family was being subjected to the "36-hour day" of caring for a dementia patient. I still have twinges of guilt now and then and always will but know that placing Charlie in a care facility was best for both of us. Not that all of my problems were over; they were just different ones.

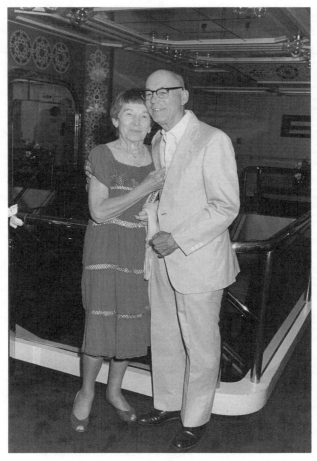

Carol and Charlie while on board the
Mississippi Queen Steamboat

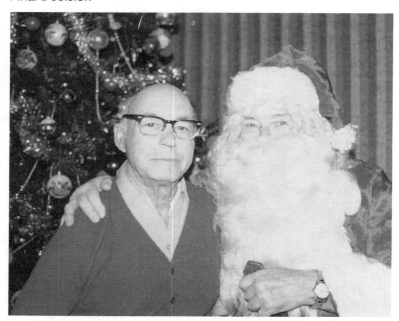

Charlie With Santa Claus, Christmas 1986,
in a Nursing Home.

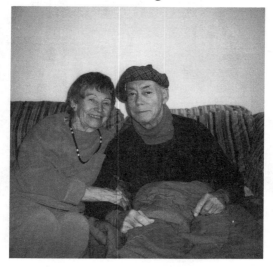

Carol visiting Charlie at Christmas,1989,
in a Nursing Home.

Seven

LIFE IN CARE FACILITIES

Ask, and it shall be given unto you; seek, and ye shall find; knock, and it shall be opened unto you.

Matthew 7:7

Having Charlie at Rosewood did not mean that my worries were over. Even though I knew I had made the right decision, guilt feelings overwhelmed me. My first husband Walter died suddenly two days before Christmas from a massive aneurysm of the lower aorta. The shock and pain were almost unbearable, but one has to accept death. I found that having Charlie as a husband and yet not as a husband was even more difficult than losing Walter.

Several weeks passed tranquilly. Just when I felt that Charlie was adjusting to his new living arrangements, I received a phone call from Gwen at Rosewood informing me that he had been missing since ten that morning. I glanced at the clock, which showed the time to be twelve-thirty. Alzheimer patients do wander. Rosewood cannot legally lock them in but makes every effort to see that a responsible person is with them when they venture out.

Charlie had gone for a stroll with Alex, who has diabetes and walks with a slow gait. Unfortunately, when Alex turned back, Charlie took off. By the time Alex returned to Rosewood, Charlie was out of sight. Some of the staff drove around trying to find him. Gwen alerted the sheriff's office. I called our local police department and remained at home in case Charlie arrived there.

About eight that evening, Gwen phoned, saying that Mr. Austen, a concerned citizen, and his wife found Charlie leaning against a light post in front of the post office in our town and took him to the police station. A policeman returned him to Rosewood. Gwen did not want me to come over until the next day but did permit me to talk with him on the phone.

> Charlie: "Honey, it's so hard to be lost and not know what to do. I knocked on peoples' doors, but no one would let me in."
>
> Carol: "Charlie, many people are afraid to open their doors to strangers."
>
> Charlie: "I know that, but I'm not a stranger."

I phoned Mr. Austen to express my gratitude for his actions. He asked, "Does Charlie have Alzheimer's? He was so disoriented he could not tell us his name." I told Mr. Austen that Charlie had identification in his wallet, to which he responded, "I was afraid to ask him for a wallet, for fear he would think we wanted to rob him."

That night tears wet my pillow when I thought of how my poor darling must have suffered. The next morning Charlie remembered nothing about his experience. We never did learn how he managed to arrive at the Camarillo post office, a distance of about fifteen miles from Rosewood. He had been a postal service employee for thirty years. We surmised that some motorist had picked him up and Charlie requested that he be taken there.

Despite the above experience, there were many pleasant hours at Rosewood. Family night was celebrated once a month. Sometimes a band played dance tunes for those who could participate. Charlie loved dancing. With his ailment and shuffling walk, once the band started to play songs of the twenties and thirties, he was up on the floor, swinging me around with as much vigor as in our high school days. Over the past few years, he had learned more modern dances, including rock, but could not remember any of them. I thought this very strange, but our doctor told me that the portion of the brain which controls dancing had not been affected. I still enjoyed the waltzes, fox trots, polkas, and, of course, the Charleston, which he remembered.

Charlie found friends in the home, who, like him, were Alzheimer patients. He even found a girl friend. At first I was jealous. Then I realized that if I could no longer be with him, I should be happy that he found someone else in whom he could become interested. He was beginning not to know me even though I was there almost every day.

When I attended one family night, I found Charlie sitting in the front row, holding the hand of a very attractive woman, named Helen. My first thought was "Dear God, I've lost my husband." Then reason prevailed. Wasn't it wonderful? If I could not be with him all the time, I wanted him to have all the happiness he could find.

I learned that Helen was a former ballet dancer. She was a tiny vivacious lady, who appeared to be many years younger than her actual age of eighty-five. She also has Alzheimer's.

Another day when I visited Charlie, he said, "See that girl over there. She's my wife, and we're going to have a baby."

Eight months later, Charlie did not recognize his own children. He was always delighted to see me. One day he tried to introduce me to a new friend by saying,

"This is...." Then, turning to me, "What are you?"

"I am Carol, and I am your wife."

"Oh, that's what I've been trying to think of."

When Ted and Evelyn, our next-door neighbors, visited Charlie at Rosewood, he became the proud host, taking them on a tour of the facilities. As they were leaving, he said, "The food is excellent, and the best part about this place is that everything is free."

Actually, he appeared to be quite content at Rosewood. With his ready smile and contagious laugh, he made many friends. In retrospect, I felt that Rosewood was the answer for both of us.

I still missed him with all my heart. At times I shed copious tears. Then I would think of the happy memories:

...Holding hands and feeling like teenagers as we took long walks in the park or down at the ocean.

...Our wedding in the gardens of the University of California at Irvine, with which I was associated.

...The trips we enjoyed together even after we knew he had Alzheimer's.

In late January of 1987, Margaret, Charlie's stepdaughter, and her husband Cliff, drove down from their home in San Jose and took Charlie and me out for lunch. Charlie didn't seem to know them.

The next day he was waiting for me in Rosewood's lounge when I entered. He asked me about the big people.

Carol: "What big people?"

Charlie: "Up north, you know."

Carol: "They had to go home."

Charlie: "I thought they were coming with you to take me back to their place."

He sounded so disappointed that my heart ached for him.

Later in the year, Charlie broke the frame on his glasses. I took him to Kaiser's clinic in Granada Hills. He became angry when he learned that the frame could not be repaired immediately. On our way back to Rosewood, he attempted to jump out of the car.

Several weeks later, Charlie greeted me with "I'm so glad to see you, but what's your name?" He knew I was his wife, but couldn't remember my name. On my next visit, I entered singing, "Here I am! Here I am! Here's your wife Carol!"

One afternoon I took him to Thrifty's for an ice cream cone. He was very unsteady on his feet. At lunch he had dropped his napkin. While reaching down to retrieve it, he hit his mouth on the table and received a nasty bruise. His conversation was rambling and hallucinatory.

By this time, I had resumed some of my social life and volunteer activities, walked two miles most days, played golf, and enjoyed swimming in Camarillo Springs' pool. For almost a year Charlie seemed to be on a plateau. Rosewood is an intermediate care facility. If patients become incontinent or nonambulatory, their families are asked to move them.

The day finally arrived in November of 1987 when Gwen asked me to come into her office and requested that I find another home for him. He not only could not manage to diaper himself, but had removed one that a staff member had put on him and tried to flush it down the toilet. The disaster resulted in an overflow which entered

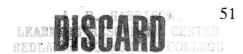

both the bath and bedroom and ruined the latter's carpeting.

The staff and many of the patients gathered around for his farewell. Most had tears in their eyes, as his good nature had endeared him to them. I shed the most tears.

We drove to Dora's Bed and Board, a private home recommended by Rosewood. It was located in a neighborhood of beautiful sprawling ranch-type dwellings with many trees. Dora and her husband Harry with their two small children, large yard, and several friendly dogs appeared to be a wonderful solution to my problem. Dora showed us Charlie's room with cheerful wallpaper, a pleasant view toward the mountains, and a television set. There were three other patients in the home. I was told that Charlie was free to roam through the house and yard and play the piano if he wished. Since this was a board and care home, naturally the monthly charge was higher — $1200.00 plus the cost of his diapers, which averaged $100.00 a month.

Two weeks later, Dora became ill and had to be hospitalized. On my next visit, I found Charlie sitting in a small bedroom with the other three women patients in wheelchairs. All seemed to be stupefied, although Dora had assured me that no tranquilizers would be administered without a doctor's prescription.

At six-thirty the next morning, my telephone rang. The receptionist at Rosewood told me that Charlie was there in nothing but his shoes and pajamas. He had been found wandering on a street in Thousand Oaks and was picked up by a man, who drove him to Rosewood, as Charlie still had their identification band on his wrist.

I immediately drove to Rosewood to get him and return him to Dora and Harry's. He didn't remember leaving their home or give me any reason for wandering.

While Charlie resided at Rosewood, I took him out for lunch or an ice cream cone several times a week. I continued the practice at Dora and Harry's. Several days after Dora's departure Harry gave Charlie's room to a woman, who came in to help keep house and care for the patients. He assured me that it would be Charlie's again when she returned. I thought if we could be patient, everything would eventually be settled to our satisfaction.

Harry was reluctant to tell me where Dora was hospitalized. I finally received the name of the hospital from the new woman of the house. I phoned there. The "hospital" turned out to be a rehabilitation center for alcoholics and drug addicts. Now I wondered if she might be gone for months.

My worries about the present situation were confirmed the next time I took Charlie to Thrifty's for an ice cream cone. He always made the same request, "When are you going to take me home with you?" I kept telling him that I still needed more rest. This time there was an added urgency in his voice. As we pulled up in front of the house, Charlie panicked. He turned to me and shouted, "Don't take me back in there. I'd rather be dead." With those words he crawled over the seat and curled up on the floor of the car. He couldn't tell me what was wrong, but I felt there was more to it than appeared on the surface.

What should I do next? The obvious solution would be to go in the house, confront Harry, and remove Charlie's belongings. But what then? I left Charlie on the floor of the back seat after telling him he did not have to live there any longer, but that I had to go in to get his clothes and toilet articles.

Harry was upset but did help me collect everything.

I phoned Gwen to tell her our latest saga. She had no idea that Dora had a problem.

During the previous two weeks, I investigated a number of other care homes in Ventura County. No vacancies at any of the good ones. The manager of Oxnard Manor on Gonzales Road asked me if I was aware of Rossiter, a new facility, opening shortly, geared to handle only Alzheimer patients. I immediately drove over there, was impressed with the manager and surroundings, and put in an application for Charlie. I was shocked at the monthly charge which increased to $2100 ($25,200 a year), including diapers. I knew I couldn't afford this amount for long, but I had little choice. Opening day happened to be exactly one week away from Charlie's outburst.

I wondered if Rosewood would take Charlie back during the interval. Gwen was reluctant but finally said that they could handle him in the daytime, but I would have to get a nurse or nurse's aide at night. Since the financial burden of Charlie's care had depleted our bank account to an alarming degree, and the minimum I would have to pay would be $11.75 an hour for seven twelve-hour shifts, I asked if she would permit me to be the caregiver at night. I stayed with him from seven p.m. to seven a.m., then went home to sleep eight hours during the day. Believe me, the nurse or aide would have been worth it.

The day finally arrived for Charlie to enter Rossiter. On November 15 of 1987, we drove from Thousand Oaks to Ventura. Flora, the administrator, showed him around and permitted him to choose his own room, which opened onto a large atrium. Blue is his favorite color. Sturdy oak chests and night stands and blue drapes and bedspreads gave a warm welcome to Charlie and his roommate George, who was a delightful person in the first stages of Alzheimer's.

During the next few weeks, I felt that a great burden had been lifted from my shoulders, although I still devoted about twenty hours a week taking him to the doctor, podiatrist, or dentist, running errands, and making round trips to see him.

Only five patients were admitted on opening day. Rossiter wanted to build up its clientele gradually to the forty-nine bed capacity.

In December, Charlie's son, Sam, two of his five children, and Henri, Charlie's ex-wife, visited from Northern California. Charlie said, "I'm so glad to see you. What's your name? What's your name? You haven't been to see me for such a long time, I thought you were dead." All of us went to Carrow's restaurant for lunch. It was a great day for Charlie.

I remained until bedtime. He stood in the middle of the room, not seeming to know what to do. He asked me, as he had once before, "What should I do with my shoes, take them off or leave them on for the night," I replied, "You will sleep better without them." I helped him remove the shoes and tucked him into bed.

At that time, Charlie's table manners were still acceptable. He enjoyed going out for meals and concerts, which were held on the first Sunday of every month in Thousand Oaks.

Activities and entertainment abounded at Rossiter. Games were played in the atrium. Charlie liked throwing the basketball into a hoop erected about four feet from the ground. Different volunteer groups sang, played instruments, and joined in games with the patients. On Saturday nights a live band performed for the dancers. To my amazement, the first time I visited one of these affairs I saw Charlie grab the activities' director and swing her around the floor to the music of a fast polka.

During the month of December, carolers strolled through the halls singing Christmas songs. Charlie sang all of the words along with them. He proudly showed me paper chains on the Christmas tree in the lounge, some of which he had made.

One day I took an album, containing pictures of Charlie in his youth, to show Mary, the wife of another Alzheimer sufferer. She commented on how good-looking he appeared at the age of twenty-eight. After months of Charlie not wanting to look at any of his albums, he looked at the picture and said, "Yes, that is a good-looking man," not realizing it was he. Then he glanced at another photo of four people and said, "That's my sister, mother, father, and my uncle," making a correct assessment.

As I was leaving Rossiter that day, Charlie walked to the door with me and said, "You can't walk out. It isn't fair. Do you think if I told them I lost my keys and couldn't get in, they would let me go home with you?" I answered, "I'm sorry, darling. Be patient a little longer."

Another day he announced, "My mother and father haven't visited me for a long time. I know they don't have any money. Where can I get some to send them?" "Charlie," I said, "The reason they haven't visited you is because they died years ago." He seemed to understand and replied, "Oh, that's too bad."

In January of 1988, I took Charlie to the podiatrist and brought him to our home for lunch. I found him standing at the kitchen sink holding a knife with the inside pockets of his slacks pulled out. "What are you doing?" I asked. "I'm cutting it out," he replied. He had left some Kleenex in his pants, and I had put them in the washing machine without realizing it. Instead of picking the shreds left, he was going to cut the whole pocket away.

The day I was dreading arrived. Rossiter's administrator Flora called me into her office and said that they could not keep Charlie much longer since his legs showed signs of becoming nonambulatory. Originally Rossiter planned to keep patients until they died or withdrew. Those plans did not materialize.

Again I called Ventura County's care homes and found that the situation was even worse than the previous year with long waiting lists.

Two weeks passed. Charlie and I went out for our usual enjoyable ice cream cone. I had prayed many times since my conversation with Flora. I asked God to help us again. I know that he did because of the next incident.

After returning to Rossiter's parking lot, I was helping Charlie get out of the car when an attractive woman in her late thirties approached us. Charlie's face lit up as she looked at him fondly and said, "Charlie and I are old friends." Thus did I meet Paulette. If I had been five minutes sooner or five minutes later, our paths would not have crossed.

Paulette had been working part time at Rossiter as a physical therapist and masseuse, but I had never met her. She said that she came over to say "goodbye" to Charlie as she had just turned in her resignation. I asked what her future plans were. Her answer: "Take one patient into our home." I told her about Flora requesting that I find a new place for Charlie and asked if she would consider him. She seemed delighted. Result: I visited their comfortable middle-class home, which she shares with Rob, her husband, who is a former teacher at the Will Rogers school across the street, but now operates a small nursery school in their home. They agreed to take Charlie for $1800 a month plus diapers.

On September 6, 1988, Charlie had a wonderful new abode, complete with two large dogs and six nursery school children, whose mothers brought them to Paulette and Rob for day care and some school lessons. One of the dogs, Sheba, immediately adopted Charlie, sat at his feet in the living room, and slept on the floor next to his bed at night.

Charlie became a member of the family. Paulette and Rob took him in his wheelchair to visit relatives and friends, on shopping trips, and out for lunch.

Several weeks passed. I began to relax. Alas! The phone rang. Paulette said that Charlie ran out of the house. She followed and was amazed at his agility as he tried to scale their six-foot fence. She and Rob brought him back into their home with difficulty. I, also, was amazed as the previous Sunday my brother Ralph, his wife Alice, and I took Charlie out for lunch. He needed support from Ralph on one side and me on the other side for him to barely drag his feet along the sidewalk. Alzheimer patients sometimes exhibit superhuman strength.

I went over the next morning. Charlie seemed to understand when I asked him if he liked living there and if Paulette and Rob were good to him. He answered "Yes" to both questions. There was no recollection of the previous evening.

The following day, Paulette phoned, saying "Charlie went berserk last night. He knocked his television set off its stand, turned over a table, and broke a chair." I phoned our doctor, who prescribed Haldol. Charlie became hyperactive and frustrated. Back to the doctor's office. He added Halcione. The two medications appeared to calm him down.

Charlie maintained a wonderful relationship with the nursery school children, who arrived each morning through the week. They called him "Uncle Charlie," which delighted him. At first I couldn't understand why they loved him so much. Then it dawned on me that here was an adult, who smiled at them all the time, listened to their chatter even though he didn't understand what they were saying, never told them what to do, and never scolded them.

Six months of comparative peace passed. Feelings of relief swept over me as life became almost normal.

But: Life has its "ups and downs."

One of the "Downs."

On March 6, 1991, Paulette phoned that evening to tell me that Rob was filing for divorce and asked her to move out. I knew they were having problems, but thought they were minor ones. Paulette said, "I'm taking Charlie to a neighbor's home for the night." I felt utterly miserable with a bad case of the flu, but made numerous telephone calls the next morning to board and care homes I had previously investigated. When I reached Felicia, a Filipino lady in the Simi Valley, she agreed to take Charlie on a trial basis for $1400.00 a month.

Paulette helped me move him in the afternoon. It was 26 miles to pick up Charlie and Paulette, then another 65 miles to drop Charlie off and return to her home. By the time I reached my home, I was exhausted.

Felicia lives in an upper middle class neighborhood. Her lovely 3,000 square foot home was tastefully decorated with fine oriental furniture. All rooms, including five bedrooms and four baths, were spacious and airy. Four women patients shared the home. I was dubious about Felicia handling Charlie, as she is no longer young and is petite. He could not take care of himself except sometimes he can hold a spoon with his right hand, shove food onto it with his left hand, and carry it to his mouth. The upper portion of his body was still strong, but he had to be lifted from bed to wheelchair or bathroom.

After two weeks, Felicia said that she was not strong enough to care for him, but she referred me to a friend of hers, Maria, who also has a board and care home with three fairly active men as patients. Maria is a strong husky woman in her middle 30s.

Three days passed. I visited each day and realized that Charlie needed a full nursing home. He had been on waiting lists at five of them for a couple of years. My daughter Susan said, "Mom, you are never going to get him in one of them. You want him to go in as a MediCal patient. As long as the homes have paying patients, they will not accept MediCal ones, as the state does not reimburse the nursing homes as much money as they receive from paying patients."

I decided to investigate Thousand Oaks Healthcare Center, which is only a mile from our home. A patient in a three bed room had died that morning. The administrator Marilyn was looking at a waiting list as I entered. I appealed to her on a compassionate level, saying that Charlie would be out on the street if he did not get into a nursing home. She agreed to take him. The monthly fee was $90.50 per day plus incidentals. I didn't ask what a private room would be, but learned later that a two-bed room is $100.00 a day. That is approximately $36,000 per year. Some of the incidentals include: $25 for monthly doctor's visits, $25 for laundry, extra personal care, beauty, and hair services, etc. Charlie is now in his new home. I don't believe that he even knew that he had been moved. He sits in a wheelchair most of the day sound asleep. As a safety measure, he has to be strapped in. When he is awake, he chafes at the support and tries to tear if off. He will babble some words to me, which I think mean that he wants me to remove it — extremely frustrating for both of us. While he is nonambulatory, his upper body is remarkably strong. The other day he tried to get out of the wheelchair. In the process, both he and the wheelchair overturned. The doctor examined him and said there were no bruises, and he seemed fine. However, Charlie was so angry that he lashed out at the nurses. The doctor prescribed a mild tranquilizer. Since that time he seems calm and relaxed. I visit almost every day and feed him one of his meals. Most of the time, his eyes stay closed, but he keeps his mouth open for me to fill it. The food looks so good that I wish I could have some for myself.

One of the "Ups."

No matter how depressing a nursing home may be, there are many touching and humorous incidents. The tender loving care accorded many of the patients by their sons or daughters is a revelation to see after reading about elder abuse.

One day when I visited, I found Charlie sound asleep in his wheelchair. I have become friendly with the wife of the patient in the next bed. He is a professor emeritus from

California Lutheran University, where he taught English and Creative Writing. His name is also Charlie. His wife Ber (Bernice) told me that a Japanese program was being offered in the dining hall. I wheeled Charlie, still sound asleep, down there. A Japanese lady, who doesn't speak English, was making paper hats and birds to give to the patients, some of whom seemed quite alert. A Japanese interpreter told the audience about origami, the traditional art of folding paper to make birds, animals, and flowers. Haunting Japanese tunes played in the background while a bird in a cage offered his own musical notes.

The flower lady came over to Charlie, who was half awake by this time, and put a flower in his hand. Like a small baby, he immediately tried to eat it.

The program ended. As I turned to leave with Charlie, I heard a magnificent rendering of "Ave Maria" floating over the room. The sound came from a beautiful, petite woman in a wheelchair. Her silvery hair fell over her shoulders in a cascade of waves. I asked the man I assumed to be her husband if she had ever been in opera, to which he replied, "Yes, she was with the New York Opera Company for years."

The above story demonstrates another strange but true feature of Alzheimer's. Long after the rest of memory and speech are gone, patients can still sing and play the piano or other musical instruments. Music taps into long term memory, requires little control from a leader or the patient and is a wonderful group activity. I remember about two years ago, Paulette told me that Charlie kept saying "sticks, sticks, sticks." She didn't know what he meant but gave him two forks. He immediately began "playing the drums." Paulette said his rhythm was great.

After I returned Charlie to his room, I walked toward the exit. On the way I was stopped by a man in a wheelchair. In a business-like tone, he asked, "Would you like to buy some stock today?" I had difficulty smothering a burst of laughter.

Some days Charlie recognizes me but doesn't know my name or that I am his wife — only that in some way I belong to him.

I wish I could know what his thoughts are. I can sense his feelings of frustration by the way he doubles up his fists and flails them in the air.

I wonder how he really felt when the doctor told him that he could no longer drive.

I wonder if he is afraid that I will forsake him, or does he no longer care?

I wonder about the anger inside him when attendants, male and female, give him a shower.

I wonder what the future will bring but know that with love and assistance we can manage.

Reality

The reality of our situation is that due to the federal rulings on Medicaid, I was informed that I had too much money (meager as it was) and would have to "spend down" or spend a goodly portion before Charlie can be approved for Medicaid or MediCal. To obtain money to pay for Charlie's nursing home care, I had to sell my home and at age 78 move in with my daughter. I will soon be impoverished because of no provision within the U. S. Medicare program to provide funding for nursing home care for Alzheimer's or other dementia type patients. To salvage some of our savings, I received legal advice that I should go to Mexico to obtain a divorce from Charlie. Not a predicament that I liked.

PART II

WHAT TO DO?

Eight

HOME HEALTH CARE

Charity is a thing that begins at home and usually stays there.

E. Hubbard

In the process of caring for Charlie, I made lots of mistakes, but I also learned from my experience and reading literature about the disease and dementia. Suggestions are made in Part II that can help you to understand the problems and ease the troubled path ahead.

Most individuals try to keep their loved one in a home setting as long as possible to preserve their happiness. You will probably have this desire too. The trend to keep elderly persons with Alzheimer's and other dementia diseases in their own homes with some type of outside assistance is popular in the United States, as well as other countries. Medicare will now pay towards home nursing assistance. Check with your social security office to find out what is available in your area.

In Europe and Canada, visiting nurses and also doctors make house calls to the home-bound elderly. There are many possible solutions to consider prior to admitting your loved one to a full-time nursing home.

THE PHASES OF ALZHEIMER'S DISEASE

The course of Alzheimer's disease has been divided into four phases. We can all recognize some of these symptoms in ourselves, but they are generally the result of fatigue, illness, or depression, and we recover. You will want to consider what phase your spouse or loved one is in when determining to keep him or her at home as long as possible. The Alzheimer's disease patient can be described as follows.

FIRST PHASE - The individual is less spontaneous, slower. They have less energy and drive. They are less discriminating, suffer a loss of words, are slower to learn and slower to react. They readily become angry and seek the familiar, which they prefer. Often this phase is insidious and no one is absolutely sure anything is wrong.

SECOND PHASE - The person is much slower in speech and understanding. They have great difficulty in making decisions and plans. They cannot calculate, become increasingly self-absorbed and insensitive to the feelings of others. They avoid situations that lead to failure. At this stage, while the individual is still functioning in many ways, the patient may need supervision in specialized activities such as balancing a checkbook.

THIRD PHASE - The patients show markedly changed behavior. They are uncertain as to how he or she is expected to act. Directions need to be repeated. The memory of recent past is poor and failing, while the long term memory of the distant past becomes astonishingly clear. The individual may invent words, misidentify people. They become lethargic and show little warmth. At this phase, the patient is obviously disabled.

FOURTH PHASE - The Alzheimer's patient becomes apathetic, displays poor remote or recent memory. They cannot find their way around at all and may become incontinent. There is no recognition of individuals. In this phase, help is needed with simple activities of daily living.

Progression of mental and physical deterioration may be rapid or it may proceed slowly over a number of years. Listed below are some alternative considerations that you may want to look into prior to choosing a full time nursing home for your loved one.

MEALS ON WHEELS

At first, all that may be necessary to relieve the caregiver is to have home meal deliveries, available in many communities. Before Charlie developed Alzheimer's, he and I took Meals On Wheels to house-bound individuals, making it possible for them to have a good, nourishing lunch. Some even ordered a light supper. The cost is nominal. To my knowledge, no one is ever turned away due to lack of funds.

HOME HEALTH CARE

Many times a person may be better off at home if outside assistance is available. Home Health Care provides nursing in the home through Visiting Nurses' Associations. Check with your Health and Social Services organizations to find out what is available in your area. Some costs are covered under Medicare.

Many helpful devices, such as canes, walkers, wheelchairs, crutches, etc., are available. I obtained a wheelchair for Charlie from our church. He was allowed free use for as long as he needed it.

ADULT DAY CARE CENTERS

These facilities give elderly persons a chance to enjoy life more fully and provide relief to the caregiver. The one in Camarillo, California, where I took Charlie, was a Godsend even if only for one day a week. Some caregivers sign up for five days a week. The cost is nominal. Transportation from home to the center is provided by many of them.

BOARD AND CARE HOMES

These are usually private facilities that furnish a room, three meals a day, and personal care services such as help with bathing, dressing, and 24-hour protection. Patients are not confined to a bed. Rehabilitation is stressed. Some offer social, recreational, and therapy programs for those who are capable of handling them. The first board and care home, in which Charlie dwelled for a year, provided trips to places of interest, took the patients out for lunch once a week, and brought in dance bands and special programs for entertainment. Crafts and games were available to those who could participate. Many have a barber and beauty shop. The Ombudsperson in your area can give you much useful information about these homes.

Often family members feel responsible for a patient with Alzheimer's disease. You may find yourself in a situation that is as bewildering to you as the disease is to the patient. You may not feel that you understand what is happening and are not equipped to deal with the enormous emotional, physical, and possible financial problems. In my search to find help for Charlie I secured a manual published by The Burke Rehabilitation Hospital Auxiliary, of White Plains, New York, entitled, *Home Management of the Person with Intellectual Loss (Dementia or Alzheimer's Disease)*.[1] It offers excellent guidelines. The four phases of Alzheimer's Disease listed above and the following suggestions are taken from that manual.

MANAGING AT HOME

Often Alzheimer's patients themselves become aware of memory loss before family and friends notice it. He or she will cover up by relying on written reminders, cueing others to mention their names first or by changing the subject.

For the person who suffers this gradual memory loss there is a devastating loss of a sense of personal dignity and a complete lack of confidence. Confusion and disorientation result in fear, anxiety, irritability, restlessness, and sleeplessness. You will need patience and understanding to handle these problems.

Because the degree of functional dependence will keep pace with the progression of the disease, it becomes necessary to continually determine how much assistance — human or mechanical — is needed to aid and protect the patient.

Matter-of-factness, repetition, consistency, and good humor will help to achieve a calm atmosphere in the home. A quiet voice is preferable. So are touching and patting, reassuring and praising, indicating affection, trust and protection. Appropriate humor is always helpful. Try to simplify routines and reduce available choices to allay frustration for both yourself and the patient.

AIDS TO MEMORY (REALITY ORIENTATION)

You can help to make the most of your loved one's residual abilities by keeping avenues of communication open; give verbal cues to help keep him or her oriented. Try to maintain a calm, normal atmosphere at home with a consistent routine. Name events on the day's schedule, repeat the names of individuals aloud, including your own.

Some useful memory aids include a large prominent clock, a large wristwatch, and a calendar with the days marked to help keep track of time. A list of the day's activities in the order of their occurrence (including mealtimes and menus) can be posted on a bulletin board or written in large letters on a sheet of paper.

Repeat instructions frequently or write them down. Keep books, magazines, and other implements of daily living in the same place all the time. Many patients enjoy looking at family photographs. The album or a box of pictures can be kept near your loved one's favorite chair.

BATHING AND GROOMING

Some people may resist bathing or changing to clean clothes. But safety, simplicity, and self-esteem are the prime considerations in grooming activities. Self-esteem accrues to the person who is clean and neatly dressed. It may become necessary to remind your relative often why bathing and changing are necessary. If they continually balk, ask your doctor to write on a prescription pad "Bath - 2 or 3 times weekly." By having this prescription on hand, it may be easier to persuade someone to bathe when he or she resists.

Only one task should be attempted at a time. Lay out the soap, wash cloth, and towel before beginning. Check the temperature of the bath or shower. Showers are generally easier. Tub bathing should only be attempted if the patient is agile enough to get in and out of the tub independently.

Remove the lock on the bathroom door. Always stay in attendance, especially when the individual is shaving or using a hair dryer. The installation of handrails, tub mats and other assistive devices are advisable as safety precautions. Use plastic instead of glass containers.

BED WETTING/INCONTINENCE

Bed wetting and incontinence are common problems with Alzheimer's patients. It was so with my husband, Charlie. When the capacity to respond to the signal or to remember where urine or feces are to be deposited is impaired, supervision becomes necessary.

Establish a toileting program by reminding the person to go to the bathroom every two hours. Use special reminders on rising in the morning, after meals, and before bedtime. Utilize special clothing designed for the incontinent adult. These can be obtained from surgical supply houses or some drug stores. Adult sized diapers, protective bedding, and disposable bed pads are also available.

You may want to restrict the intake of fluids for some hours before bedtime. Place a commode or urinal bottle near the bed. If nighttime incontinence becomes severe, you might consult your doctor about using an external catheter and collecting bag at night.

Bowel movements can be regulated through the use of enemas or suppositories. Fecal incontinence and fecal impaction may occur at a later phase. Your doctor can help you to recognize problems.

CHILDREN

Alzheimer's patients enjoy small children with their happy natures and unembarrassed manners. Don't discourage visiting and playing if there are small children in your family. At times, teenagers may be embarrassed to introduce a mother, father or other relative who does not behave normally. It is important that you explain that the patient is sick and that Alzheimer's disease is not rare. Encourage young people to bring friends home after explaining what the problem of the patient is.

COMPREHENSION

You may find it very difficult to lower your expectations of a loved one with whom you have lived closely for many years, but it becomes necessary to do so in dealing with Alzheimer's patients. Don't try to explain or make the individual do something when he or she is no longer capable of understanding. Avoid conflict by showing how a task can be accomplished and then helping them to follow your instructions. Reinforce thoughts by using pictures or gestures - e.g., by referring to the sense of smell (as with flowers) or the sense of taste. Whenever possible you can inject the situation with humor. Speak slowly, distinctly, and softly. Repeat ideas. Maintain eye contact to help the patient keep focused.

DEPRESSION

You will probably experience depression and anger when living with a relative who suffers memory loss and intellectual decline. It is to be expected. Don't let depression become severe. Seek individual or group Counseling. If you are concerned about the patient's depression, seek advice from your physician.

DRESSING

Choose simple, easy and appropriate dress. Reduce choices in color and style. Garments with front closing, large zipper pulls, and few buttons are easiest to put on. Cardigans are better than slipover sweaters. If incontinence or spilled food is a problem, try to use only wash and wear clothing.

If the patient is dressing, lay out the underwear first, then the outer clothes, then the shoes and socks. You may have to help by showing how to put the clothing on. It's best to stay in the room and supervise. If he or she wants to wear the same thing every day, don't argue. While dressing, there is an opportunity to praise the individual by commenting on how handsome or beautiful he or she is.

DRIVING A CAR

Driving an automobile can produce stress for a well person. For the Alzheimer's patient, driving has the potential for increasing anxiety and irritability. Some find it a relief to be rid of the responsiblity. Others, like my

Charlie, may fiercely resist the idea of giving up driving. To avoid a source of conflict, ask the physician to inform the patient that he or she can no longer drive. You should always be mindful of the safety of others and the legal implications involved.

EXERCISE

Exercise is important for good health for everyone. For the Alzheimer's patient, walking not only provides excellent exercise, but also seems to relieve tension. Using a rocking chair also seems to lessen tension and is a good indoor exercise. If the patient enjoys dancing, it too is helpful. Charlie enjoyed dancing for a long period of time. Music seems to have a beneficial effect. Movement of any kind is good. Even sweeping the floor or patio can be a form of exercise.

GOING OUT ALONE

You need to consider safety first when deciding whether or not to allow your loved one to go out alone. In the beginning, I didn't worry if Charlie went out because we lived in an enclosed community and knew all the nearby neighbors. But you need to have confidence that the person can reach the intended destination and find the way back.

Wandering is a well-known habit of Alzheimer's patients. If your relative tends to wander, place an identification tab around the neck or the wrist, giving name, address, and telephone number. Then, if he becomes lost, it will be possible for those he or she meets to help return the patient home.

Restless patients may find their way out of the house despite locked doors during the day or night. One way to avoid this is to move the door lock to the bottom of the door where the person may not think to look for it. Installation of a dead bolt lock is another preventive measure.

LOSING THINGS

It is common for Alzheimer's patients to lose things or hide things. You cannot expect anything to be returned to its customary place. You should remember to keep track of eye glasses, dentures, hearing aids, money, keys, etc. Personal items can be labeled for easier recognition. All things of value should be kept out of sight so they cannot be misplaced.

LEISURE ACTIVITIES

Complex games and crafts are not useful, but keep in mind that adults don't like to be treated as children. It has been found in group settings that patients enjoy simple games like shuffleboard if they are still able to play. Whatever is attempted, remember that the patient has a short attention span — no more than 30 minutes, often less — and has little creative capacity or sense of humor. Two very rewarding activities are gardening and music. Music particularly may help recall childhood events or past pleasures. If the individual is bilingual, music and songs which involve the first language are wonderful.

MEALTIMES

You may find mealtimes difficult, so again, try to keep them simple. Serve meals of normal nutritional value as there are no special nutritional requirements. If the patient wishes to eat one food, such as ice cream, several times a day, don't try to force him not to. Just be aware that extreme excesses can lead to excessive weight gain. If the patient is a poor eater, consider supplementing the meal with a balanced liquid drink such as "Ensure." It is better to allow a patient to eat what he or she wants rather than to not eat at all.

Announce ahead of time what the next meal is to be (breakfast, lunch, snack, dinner) and what time it will be served. Present one course at a time at the table. When one dish is finished, offer the next. You will find it necessary to become tolerant of poor table manners. Use finger foods and sandwiches when possible. Sometimes you may have to remind the patient to swallow or cut foods into small pieces for him or her. Conversation during mealtime will help create a social atmosphere. The patient should be given as many opportunities to join in the discussion as feasible.

MEDICAL CARE AND MEDICATIONS

Depending on the phase of your loved one's illness and their physical health, you will probably need to supervise medications. It is unwise to trust a forgetful person with the responsibility for administering his or her own drugs. Close collaboration between the family and the doctor is important in the prescription of medications and monitoring any adverse effects. Again, it helps to repeat to the patient what the medication is and why it is being taken when the dose is given.

NIGHTTIME SUPERVISION

Some patients sleep during the day and are awake and restless at night. Nocturnal wandering accompanied by confusion and blurred images are both disruptive and dangerous. Some medication may need to be prescribed to insure sleeping at night. If possible, try to keep the patient up during the day, discouraging napping.

If there is restlessness at night, you can try to convey feelings of comfort and security with an embrace, a back rub, and soothing words. Drawn window shades will keep the room dark during seasons of early morning light.

Precautions can include closing bedroom doors whenever feasible, and keeping a night light burning. If the person is likely to try to leave the home, a bell affixed to the exit door will alert the family when the door is opened. As mentioned earlier, the lock on the door exits can be moved to the bottom of the door where the person is less likely to find it.

SEXUAL BEHAVIOR

As the patient becomes less competent in other areas, his or her sexual performance may be affected. If the spouse feels sexually stimulated, he or she may need to take the initiative by taking a larger role in the act. Aberrant sexual behavior, such as publicly masturbating or touching others, should be gently but firmly discouraged.

SMOKING AND DRINKING

If either smoking or drinking has been a habit with a patient, it may be just as well to let the practice continue, but unwise to encourage it. Smoking should be supervised because of the danger of burns or fires. Remove cigarettes and matches if the patient is alone. Do the same if the person tends to roam the house at night.

An occasional drink before dinner is permissible, but since the mixture of alcohol and any drugs the patient may be taking can have an adverse effect, drinking should be strictly limited. The individual may not be able to judge or measure the amount of alcohol to be added to a drink, so you will need to supervise the mixing and serving of cocktails. Bottles of alcohol should be kept out of sight.

SAFETY

Boiling water, hot fat or grease, stove burners, matches, cigarette lighters, firearms, etc. all are potentially dangerous to the Alzheimer's or dementia patient. Some will drink any liquid they see. Cleaning fluids, cooking ingredients, paint supplies, etc. should be kept out of the way.

Problems with mobility may become evident, necessitating an increased awareness of extension cords, footstools, scatter rugs, and similar objects which can cause a fall. Keep household furnishings in the same place all the time in an effort to avoid accidents as well as lessen confusion.

SPEECH

Do not discourage rambling or incoherent speech, or your relative may become more and more reluctant to talk. Nod and smile while he or she is talking, and at the same time try to get the sense of the thought. Because memory of past events can be very clear, the individual may sometimes be talking about something that happened many years ago, and has suddenly interjected the thought into the current conversation. Cue the person who is fumbling for a word.

TELEPHONE

If you leave the patient alone, you may want to disconnect the telephone or attach an automatic answering device to record messages. Often a patient will answer the telephone when alone and may become upset themselves or upset the caller. It is best that telephone conversations be supervised and that an answering machine be used to answer the phone if the patient is alone for a period of time.

SOCIAL SITUATIONS

A trip to an unknown place, surrounded by strangers, sleeping and eating in unfamiliar rooms tends to upset Alzheimer's patients. There is much more comfort and ease at home where people are familiar, the location of the bathroom is known, where one is not required to order from a menu, and where magazines and the television are always in the same place.

Some success has been reported by families who have rented apartments or houses in vacation areas. They say they have been able to simulate a home-like setting and keep daily routines simple and familiar.

If the caring members of the family need a vacation, it may be desirable to leave the patient at home in a familiar place with familiar companions. Provide a reassuring note stating where you are going and when you will return.

Encourage friends and neighbors (in small numbers) to visit if they are aware of the situation and seem to be able to handle it. Repeat their names often. At social gatherings, you can supply gentle cues as reminders to the patient. Remember that many are happy to be only observers in social situations.

DAY CARE CENTERS

An interim step between caregiving in the home and institutionalization is the day care center for demented patients. When day-to-day activities can no longer be performed by the patient and both he and the caregiver experience great frustration as a result, it's time for the patient to be in a group setting with professional caregivers. In a day center setting activities are planned which maximize the patient's remaining functions. According to the experts at the Ethel Percy Andrus Gerontology Center at the University of Southern California, "The stages of the disease, ranging from loss of recent memory in the earliest stage to loss of physical functioning, speech and all memory in the latter stage, necessitate careful choice of program to stimulate and maintain functioning levels while providing the opportunity for social interaction and satisfaction." This is too much for you to provide for your loved one in your home, so if a day care center is available, it would be wise to look into what they have to offer.

Screening The Day Care Center

Questions to bear in mind are whether there is daily provision for reality orientation, social interaction, meaningful tasks at the level of his ability, sensory stimulation, and companionship with the opportunity for making friends. If these kinds of challenges are offered, matched to the capabilities of the patient, it slows the rate of deterioration. Rewards are needed, but not achievement rewards. Recognition, fleeting pleasure, hugs, and a sense of well-being are the reinforcements.

Do the staff appear to be knowledgeable about the disease? Do they offer enough control to provide the participants with a feeling of security without being over-controlling? Are directions given slowly and clearly? Is participation encouraged? Do they have a reasonable schedule of planned and supervised events? If so you are fortunate indeed to have such a resource to tide you over until your loved one needs nursing home care.

COMMUNITY RESOURCES

Caregivers are at risk of becoming depressed because of isolation and loneliness. It is easy to fall into that trap especially if independence is one of your values, and it's difficult for you to ask for help. You may need to remind yourself that it is a high level coping skill to make use of appropriate resources. Resources do exist for people in your position and it makes good sense for you to make connections with them — whether it's the Alzheimer's Hot Line (1-800-272-3900) or a local support group.

A support group is one which you can count on for non-judgmental acceptance and encouragement, and that will keep your discussion in confidence. It is a place to gain information, coping skills, and emotional support. Other people who are in the same position as you, suffering the same pain and frustration, can be an enormous help in alleviating your loneliness, too.

You will find a listing of specific National Resources in Part III, but in general, the following is a list of the kinds of community agencies that either provide resources that you need, or can direct you to a support group, or other kind of help you are seeking. You will want to start with your local Alzheimer's Organization, but in addition there are:

Social Service Agencies:

Your local Department of Social Services, or Welfare Department, usually will have an information and referral service.

Health Agencies:

County Health Departments, County Mental Health Departments, and Visiting Nurses Associations have educational materials and can guide you in the right direction. The social service departments of hospitals are invaluable resources.

Religious Organizations:

More and more churches and temples have social service departments that offer help. Catholic Charities, Jewish Family Service Agencies, and Protestant and non-denominational Family Agencies, are appropriate places to turn for counseling and information.

Other Resources for Special Needs:

Day Care Centers for Seniors may be under the auspices of any of the above. For legal questions look for Gray Law offices or legal aid societies. Check into County or State Offices on Aging.

Don't put off getting help, even if you feel you're too tired to make the effort. If your house were on fire you would not hesitate to call the fire department. Being an Alzheimer family is an analogous crisis even if the conflagration is not as apparent. You deserve the assistance that your national and local communities have set up to meet your need, and you have a responsibility to yourself and to your loved one to seek it out.

Nine

NURSING HOMES: CHOOSING AND LIVING IN ONE

Keep your face to the sunshine and you cannot see the shadow.

Helen Keller

As with me, the day may come when you find it necessary to put your loved one into a long-term care home. You may have said that you would never, never place him or her in one, but when the burden becomes more than you can handle, you know you have to find a solution.

WHEN TO PLACE

For the person living in a family setting, the question of placement often arises when the patient's behavior begins to have an adverse effect on the lives of other family members. Dr. James A. Haycox, M.D., former director of psychiatric services at The Burke Rehabilitation Center, writing in The New England Journal of Medicine, describes the circumstances which can influence a family to seek nursing home care for a relative:

"...It is a difficult judgement to make as to when the demented person is better cared for by professional help in a nursing home than in his own home. I believe there is a set of relative criteria and an absolute set which guide these decisions."

Dr. Haycox goes on to discuss the need to concede that the ill person can no longer do what is necessary for daily living. Social life becomes constricted, and favorite activities, even sexual enjoyment which is incapacitated by dementia, are lost. Finally the burden becomes too much for the caregivers and members of the family. "...There is an absolute criterion which nearly always dictates the decision to relinquish home care. With advancing disease there may come a time when the people are less important to the patient than the service which they give. It may no longer matter who gives the service as long as it is done, and there is no special reaction to the loved one. In the end, a patient may prefer to lie in bed undisturbed by people though he may need to be turned, bathed, and otherwise cared for. The physical needs and their satisfaction are nearly the only things that matter. At that point, a nursing home is preferable. ...I submit that the patient is safer and more content with the specialist than with the family when people are no longer perceived as individuals by him."

You will need to decide whether or not the care in a good nursing home will be more beneficial to the patient than the type he was being given at home. If you are the primary caregiver, it is very important to consider whether or not your own health and mental stability are being threatened.

HOW TO SELECT THE RIGHT PLACE

It takes time to select a good nursing home for a patient with Alzheimer's or similar disease, so here again, pre-planning is important. Be sure to consider what the advanced needs of the ill person will be, so you will not have to move them as the illness progresses. Nursing homes will handle patients in different stages of the disease and it is traumatic to both the spouse or family and the patient to have to be relocated.

NURSING HOMES

Now begins the difficult task of looking for one. Much bad publicity has been in the news about the abuses of patients, poor food, and lack of personal care. However, there are many good homes available. The term "nursing home" is actually a very general name for several types of medical-care facilities. Years ago nursing homes were not for very ill patients - the answer was a hospital. Now many of the duties formerly performed in a hospital have been taken over by nursing homes. A list of sources of help for the family is included in the Appendix.

There are two types of homes: First, skilled nursing care for people who need 24-hour-a-day supervision by a registered nurse, under the direction of a physician, who is available for emergencies if not actually on the premises; and second, intermediate nursing care for those who require some nursing assistance.

Residents are served by nursing staff at three levels: registered nurse, licensed practical nurse, who takes care of the less skilled nursing tasks, and the nursing assistant, who provides around 90 percent of the actual care given. Depending on the size of the institution, there may be rehabilitative and therapy services. Diapers, special beds, wheelchairs, laundry, etc. may not be covered in the daily rate. Some homes provide for podiatry and pharmaceutical needs, even hairdressing, for an extra fee.

Try to pick a nursing home where the patient will have friends and possibilities for developing interests, such as a library or his church nearby. Life for the elderly can be a series of losses, and to adjust well there needs to be the means of compensating for those losses in their new environment. They need social and recreational activities as well as privacy. Libraries and chapels often help with this need if private rooms are not available.

Church homes have been in existence for many years. They started out as regular retirement homes with a wing for short-term illnesses. Now many of them have extended care. While they usually have long waiting lists, they are worth waiting for.

Before looking for a home, it is important to evaluate the needs of the person entering. What suits one individual may not fit into the life style of another. Also, the financial situation of the person needs to be considered. (See Chapter Eleven on Insurance and Chapter Twelve on Legal Aspects.)

In choosing a home, take advantage of suggestions from friends, your doctor, clergyperson or priest, minister or Rabbi. The decision should not be made by any single person. It is too burdensome for one individual alone. If possible, discuss the homes long before it is necessary to place a person there. Many nursing homes are filled to their limits and may have long waiting lists. Spouses or children need time to think about placement, but occasionally emergencies arise when you need to find a nursing home that will take the patient within a few days.

If a patient goes to a nursing home directly from a hospital, social services' staff at the hospital will assist you. They will recommend several nursing homes and will help with the paperwork. They cannot choose one for you.

Preparing the Patient

Talk all of what you have learned over with your loved one if possible. From what I had read or heard since placing my husband in a care home, I made a bad mistake by telling him, "I am all worn out from taking care of you. I need a good long rest." I realized later that this was definitely the wrong way to approach the subject because for months, he kept asking me if I was rested enough to bring him home. It is better to be honest, and say something like "You need more care than I can provide. I think you'll be better off with. . . because they can give you the special services that meet your needs."Then name those needs specifically.

If the patient is lucid, be sure to engage him in all phases of the placement. Sometimes they will be angry; sometimes they know they need one and may even suggest it.

SCREENING THE HOME

Do the initial screening over the telephone, as visiting the homes is a long drawn-out procedure, which you may find unpleasant. Try to find one near the patient's neighborhood, so that friends and nearby relatives may visit often. List all of the nursing homes in the area. This may be obtained from Social Security and your local library. When you phone, ask the following questions:

1. What restrictions are there for being accepted?

2. How many patients do you have? The larger the facility, usually the more services are provided.

3. Is your home licensed or certified by the state, whose agents regularly inspect the premises?

4. Is the administrator licensed? If you receive a negative answer, don't pursue it.

5. What level of care is provided?

6. Do you accept Medicare or Medicaid?

7. Is there a vacancy? If not, how long is the waiting list?

8. What are the charges? What is included? What is extra?

9. Are special services available?

10. In an emergency, to what hospital would the doctor send the patient?

11. What is the turnover in staff?

12. Who owns the home, and what is its history?

13. What is the level of training for administrative staff?

14. Is there a doctor on the premises or one on call?

Next, call the program "ombudsperson" to see if there are any complaints about the home. In some situations it's helpful to call the ombudsman program first, as they will counsel you through the whole process. You can get this information from the home administrators.

TOURING THE HOME

From your telephone replies and the recommendations of others, visit three or four that you feel will meet the patient's needs.

When you arrive, see if the outside of the building and the grounds are well kept up. When you walk in, what do you hear or smell?

Individuals who are in nursing homes today are for the most part older, sicker, and more frail than those of the past. So, don't be frightened. Be prepared to accept this.

What is your impression of the staff you are meeting? How do the residents look? Are there call bells to summon help next to the bed and in the bathroom?

How are roommates chosen? What about bathroom facilities: private or shared by others? How many nurses and nursing aides are there for each patient?

What restraints are used? Sometimes these are necessary for the safety of the patient, but they must be prescribed by a doctor; e.g., soft belts around waists in wheelchairs.

Examine the kitchen. What about snacks? Ask to see the room in which your loved one will be placed. Stop and chat with residents.

After the tour by an administrator or other dignitary, take time to go back and, on your own, inspect the home by talking to the residents and staff. Check the state survey records of the two homes you like the most. Since some homes go through a bad period, take this into account.

It would be wise to make a second visit to the home you select. You may notice other things unobserved before. Read the admissions contract and other literature provided carefully. If possible, have it reviewed by an attorney.

The best time to move in is between two and four in the afternoon. Some patients adjust rapidly; some take several weeks; some never adjust.

NURSING HOME COSTS

You will need to discuss finances. Depending on the age and physical condition of your spouse, the cumulative cost of years of nursing home care can be enormous. Some families can pay expenses from their own assets. Most cannot. Possibly, the patient is eligible for Medicaid (Medi-Cal in California). Title XIX Social Services is helpful here. It might be best also to consult an attorney who specializes in Eldercare. If this is the case, make certain that the nursing home you select will accept Medicaid persons. You may be told there is a long waiting list. Most homes prefer patients that can pay because Medicaid does not cover their costs.

The patient at this point may need to have you or some other trusted relative or friend be appointed as legal guardian or have power of attorney should he not be able to make decisions for himself. This is discussed in more detail in Chapter Eleven, Legal Aspects.

Estimate the individual's net monthly income. As of January 1990, a spouse may no longer have separate property. Everything is considered community property. This worked to my disadvantage. Charlie and I have been married for almost fourteen years. With the exception of a joint checking account, we have always kept our money separate. The assets that I accumulated before I married Charlie have always been in my former married name in trust for my children, while his were in his name in trust for his children.

Four years ago I applied for MediCal for Charlie since his savings had dwindled to his pension and social security, which in no way covered the cost of the homes. It was approved by the Public Social Services Agency. Then Charlie seemed so content where he was that I decided not to accept it and kept using my money to supplement his care, which was a serious mistake. This year I realized that I could not continue to keep on paying or I would have nothing left for my own old age. Due to the new ruling, I was informed that I had too much money (meager as it was) and would have to "spend down" or spend a goodly portion before Charlie can be approved for MediCal. This action forced me to sell my house to obtain money for Charlie's health care and move in at age 78 with my daughter. I would soon be impoverished because of an inadequate national health "un-system."

Be sure you have written papers that will let you know what the nursing home charges will be and what the extras might be. Standard services are room, meals, linens, and custodial nursing care, although this may vary from state to state. The subject of burial should be discussed with the nursing home before entrance. You will also need to take insurance information, pensions, and Social Security materials, as the home will want to copy them.

New rules are implemented often, so accept the help of others: an attorney, a friend who has had similar problems, etc.

FINANCIAL FACTORS

The costs of a long-term nursing care in the United States can be catastrophic to a family. Therefore, the costs of a nursing home will greatly influence your final selection. Even when public and church funding are used to the fullest extent possible, if the patient lives a long time, it can wreak havoc with the finances of most families. To get through the fiscal quagmire that may befall your family it's important to learn the facts about your eligibility for various funding programs in advance. Carefully analyse your personal assets and those available with the community. There may be more help available than seems at first possible. Use the following check list to ensure that you covered all bases:

Current and anticipated assets:

You may want to use your tax consultant or other financial advisor to help you in estimating your current worth, how much money you can safely put aside for medical care, and any anticipated assets. Often an intake worker at your local Department of Public Social Services can help you sort this out.

Insurance:

You should consult with your insurance agent to understand exactly what benefits you are entitled to; what you can expect.

Medicare:

At present, if the patient is adjudged to have the potential for rehabilitation, Medicare covers 150 days after a minimal co-insurance amount each day for the first eight days of care during the year.

Medicaid:

The last resort is Medicaid. You will need the assistance of a social service worker from the Department of Public

Social Services, or a private agency, to help you to apply. The rules vary from state to state. Such social workers are often good at discovering resources that you are not aware of. The application process includes proof of citizenship or legal residence, and a financial review. You may or may not be liable for your spouse's debts depending on what state you live in. You may be required to pay for nursing home care for a specific period of time before you are eligible for this help. You may have to "spend down" in order for your spouse to become eligible which puts your own financial future in serious jeopardy.

Other Potential Resources:

Be sure to take advantage of any Veterans' benefits for which the patient may be eligible. Inquire at your, or the patient's religious organization to see if they have anything to offer. Check with his labor union. The health care services situation in this country is so dire, that some social action is in order. Contact your state and national legislators and inform them of your predicament. They may offer some help. A little protest might do some good.

If all else fails, go to an advocacy group to get some ideas about what to do. See the list of possible resources in the Appendix.

LIVING IN A NURSING HOME

If both husband and wife have to be institutionalized, don't do as one son and daughter did — put them in separate rooms even though they had fought all their lives but slept in the same bed together. If they enjoy bickering, let them. Leave them alone for they have needs too — both emotional and sexual.

Be sure to mark or have tags attached to clothing and personal items. If the person is capable, have him choose his favorite photos, pillows, and possibly a favorite chair. Take clothing that can be washed. I made the mistake of taking Charlie's favorite yellow wool sweater. The home threw it in the washing machine and dryer. It would have fit a two-year old before they were through.

For dementia patients, who have trouble with buttons, clasps, or hooks, take pull-on slacks and slip-over shirts and sweaters with no buttons. Do not bring any valuable possessions, medications, or snack foods unless the home OK's it. No more than a few dollars. Some homes bank the money for residents and give it to them as needed.

Keep on evaluating his care. Try to make him comfortable. If he can't talk, possibly you could say, "Father, blink your eyes or squeeze my hand if you have any pain." Also very important is keeping your promises. If you tell him you will be there on a certain day or hour, be there. I visit at mealtimes so that I can feed Charlie.

Include his roommate, if he has one, and other residents in your conversations. If you have a dog or cat, and the home permits them, a visit from a pet may bring pleasure and cheer to the patient. Some homes even have their own resident cats or dogs.

If the patient complains, take it seriously and talk with the nursing staff. If no one helps you, go to the administrator or ombudsman.

CARE FOR THE CAREGIVER

Be prepared for belligerent behavior. You may be greeted with anger as your loved ones may feel that you are taking them there to die. Everyone in some way denies the aging process, as we are a youth-oriented society. When the older person finally realizes that he might die, he may scream, yell at you and the nursing staff, and even hit anyone near him.

You may be angry, too because this is happening to both of you.

Some homes have strict rules about visiting. You may be able to go every day, but most homes usually request that at first you stay away for several days or more to give the patient an opportunity to settle down and become adjusted to his new surroundings.

Be aware that you have to make a life of your own. Get involved and pick up the threads where you left off several years ago.

While you may have guilt feelings (I certainly did), you may find that the patient is adjusting very well. He may even be happier with other people around him than he was at home.

1. *Choosing a Nursing Home for the Person with Intellectual Loss,* The Auxiliary Burke Rehabilitation Center, 785 Mamaroneck Ave., White Plains, NY 10605

Ten

INSURANCE AND FISCAL ISSUES

*Read everything carefully. What the big black type
giveth, the spidery type may take away.*

Jane Bryant Quinn

Upon realizing that the cost of caring for a dementia or
Alzheimer's patient is high and can wipe out a family's life
savings, some seek "insurance" for protection. Be fore-
warned.

You may feel that reaching the decision to place your
spouse or loved one into a nursing home was the hardest
decision of all. Once that was over, you probably experienced some relief. Unfortunately, just at the time when
you are emotionally exhausted, other financial considerations such as insurance coverage crop up.

As individuals grow older, most reel at the thought of
contracting a debilitating disease such as Alzheimer's. Not
only does the ill person suffer a loss of dignity, but the cost
of medical care may also bring financial disaster. In some
cases, the spouse or loved one may end up in poverty as
well. Ideally, to have medical coverage in place before the

illness strikes would be best. For this reason, pre-planning of insurance needs is important.

At age 65 citizens of the United States are eligible for Medicare Insurance. After paying a basic deductible amount, Part A provides for hospital coverage and Part B pays for doctors and other medical expenses. However, Medicare pays only 80 percent of the amount approved for Part B charges. This is not enough. Most Americans must purchase supplemental insurance to help cover these costs.

Unfortunately, in the case of catastrophic illness, many have not considered insurance before the illness strikes and are caught with the tremendous expense of nursing home care. This can average between $30,000 to $40,000 per year depending on your location. In addition, many individuals do not even realize that to date Medicare does not cover long term care needs.

Both Charlie and I are covered by Medicare and its coverage is inadequate. I have sold our home and spent most of our savings providing for his care, praying for the time he will become eligible for MediCal. I have been told by the State Health workers that I must "spend down" in order to qualify and I worry about my own future. Recently, legislation was enacted that covers some of the costs of in-home care, but Medicare does not provide benefits for nursing home care. In other words, the system does not consider Alzheimer's or dementia a physical illness requiring medical attention because the majority of patients only need assistance with daily living needs such as bathing, getting dressed, and preparing meals.

My own investigation of twelve leading insurance companies elicited much confusing information when I inquired about supplemental insurance policies and Long Term Care (LTC) policies. All of the companies informed me that they did have policies covering Alzheimer's disease.

When I pressed for details about exclusions and age limits, I learned the following:

1. A person must be in good health at the time the policy is taken out. (This confirms the importance of pre-planning.)

2. The policy must be in effect two years before Alzheimer's is discovered.

3. The policy is effective until the individual reaches the age of 62 (65 in some cases).

While Alzheimer's can affect people as young as 40, most do not show signs of the disease until they are in their 60s, 70s, or 80s. What chance does one have to be covered?

Only one insurance agent gave me what I consider to be the truth. "It is 99.99 percent impossible to get coverage for Alzheimer's."

Medicaid (MediCal in California) will pay for the indigent, but in order to qualify, an individual must own nothing more than their home, an automobile, term life insurance policies, and a few thousand dollars in cash. Those with more assets must "spend down" if they are to qualify for Medicaid. As you will see in the next chapter on legal considerations, many facing long-term nursing home bills resort to giving away their assets in order to qualify.

All across America, the elderly and their families are looking to the federal government for a program that will assist the middle-class if they need nursing care for a catastrophic illness. In 1989, issues were examined by the Claude Pepper Commission (named after the late Senator). Testimony from many families facing such a crisis was heard. As one witness put it, "I do know that our older people have contributed their whole lives and they deserve to be taken care of. We are all going to be there one of these days."

There is no denying that the proposals made by the Pepper Commission would be expensive, the nursing home segment alone would cost $16 billion a year and the home care portion, $32 billion.

But it is a social problem that needs solving. Senator Jay Rockefeller (Democrat-West Virginia) summed it up when he said, "I don't think it's possible to say finally and ultimately that we are a civilized nation when so many of our people do not have this access, do not have long-term care."

CARE IN GREAT BRITAIN

Consider what is available in other countries. In Britain, the National Health Service covers a comprehensive range of medical services for all citizens, irrespective of means. Local authority handles social services and volunteers provide help and advice to the elderly and disabled. Services are provided to help the elderly live at home whenever possible, for as long as possible. Only about five percent of those over 65 live in institutional accommodations. These services include assistance from social workers, domestic help, meals in the home, sitters, night attendants and laundry services, as well as day care centers. Visiting nurses attend the elderly in their homes and doctors make house calls also. When needed, transportation is provided to day care centers or for medical help.

If it becomes necessary for individuals to move to an old age home, they pay according to their ability (a percentage of their state pension and private pension if any).

CARE IN CANADA

Canada also has a taxpayer financed, comprehensive health care system that covers hospital and doctors' services for all residents regardless of ability to pay. Institutional care for the aged and infirm is provided under provincial, municipal, or voluntary auspices. Homemaker services are in place for the elderly and disabled to foster independent living. Here too, visiting nurses and doctors play a large role in helping the elderly.

Social integration centers such as Golden Age Clubs for the elderly have been established, as well as special day care centers for dementia patients. If individuals must be institutionalized, they will be charged a percentage of their pension income, based on their financial status and ability to pay. Efforts to keep the elderly at home are a priority.

A major factor in keeping health care costs down in Canada are significantly lower administrative costs. Administration accounts for about 2.5 percent of total health costs in Canada, compared to 8.5 percent in the U.S. Under the Canadian system, with a single insurer for each provincial plan, compared to 1500 private insurers in the U.S., the costs of marketing, setting premiums, and deciding who should be covered are avoided.

CARE IN SWEDEN

Overall responsibility for the care of the elderly in Sweden rests with the state. The Swedish system of national pensions and housing allowances is designed to give the elderly financial security. Special housing is provided to help them stay in their homes as long as possible. About 92 percent of the population over 65 live in ordinary homes now. Studies show that in Sweden, as well as the U.S., the majority of individuals needing nursing homes are the very elderly in their eighties.

Home health care is stressed. Visiting nurses and doctors come to the homes of the elderly needing assistance. Services to help with cooking, shopping, laundry, and personal hygiene are available. Special day care centers have been established for the elderly with Alzheimer's and other dementias. Transportation is provided.

There are three types of nursing homes in Sweden, central homes attached to a hospital geriatric unit, local nursing homes independent of hospitals, and private nursing homes. The trend is to separate frail elderly with physical ailments who need assistance and others with long term dementia disabilities. At old age homes and long term care facilities (for dementia patients) the individuals pay different amounts. For old age homes the minimum fee is 70 percent of the national basic pension plus 80% of other income. In long term care, a pensioner receives 365 days free and is allowed to keep his or her housing allowance for his regular home for the first year. After that a patient pays SEK 55 or approximately $10.00 per day.

In the past few years, Sweden has experimented with "group dwellings" for persons with dementia. These are small housing collectives of 6 to 8 persons where individuals, each having their own room, reside and are cared for. The Swedes believe this is a more humane approach than large institutions of old people. The group dwellings are being expanded. In the late 1980s there were around 1000 persons living in group dwellings.

CARE IN JAPAN

Canada and other western European countries are not alone in experiencing the health care problems associated with an increasing elderly population. In Japan, the population of those 65 or older is now approximately 11 percent. By the year 2000, this is expected to rise to 17 percent and will surpass 25 percent by 2025. Faced with this dramatic demographic shift, Japan's health planners are approaching the problem as a national burden to help fund the country's universal health-insurance and pension systems, which are now about 41 percent of national income. This burden will rise to almost 50 percent by 2020. At present, health care for those over 70 is virtually free, but that will have to change. The government plans to double the modest $2.85 fee charged per day for a hospital stay and are considering raising the age requirement for public pensions from 60 to 65. More than 60 percent of the elderly live with children or other family now, as compared to about 10 percent in the United States.

There is a tremendous shortage of nursing homes, needed for dementia patients, in the large cities. In Tokyo, for example, there are over 1300 elderly on the waiting list for one 610-bed nursing home, part of the Tokyo Metropolitan Institute of Gerontology. There is a great need for expanded home health care services in Japan also and a shortage of younger workers willing and able to handle the challenge.

In 1989 The Ministry of Health and Welfare announced a comprehensive ten-year "Golden Plan" to augment services for the aged. This would include building more geriatric rehabilitation centers, increasing the number of physical therapists and the number of public home helpers who visit elderly in their homes. Even with this, the level of benefits for the elderly in Japan would not be as high as that which already exits in the older welfare states like Sweden and Norway where costs have increased the national burden to about 60 percent.

FINANCING OF HEALTH CARE

Citizens of Britain, Canada, and Sweden pay very high taxes for such health care benefits. Costs are enormous and are continually monitored for efficiency. While not perfect, these systems are helping the elderly stay independent as long as possible, protecting families from financial disaster, and helping prevent the loss of homes. As in the United States, between the years 2000 and 2020, the elderly population is expected to increase greatly.

The present market in America for adequate Long Term Care or LTC policies is bewildering and confusing. There are no uniform terms or definitions. It is almost impossible to compare benefits or to even understand what benefits will be paid. Tricky ways in which policies are written can set the potential for unaffordable rate increases and other policy restrictions. Beware of excessive agent commissions. When shopping for such a policy, consider the advice below offered from a survey taken by Consumer Reports in June, 1991.

- Be aware that Medicare-supplement and nursing-home insurance are two completely different products. Supplement insurance pays after Medicare coverage which does not pay for Alzheimer's or other dementia patients' custodial care. Long Term Care (LTC) policies are the ones that cover nursing home stays.

- The best protection is to plan ahead. If possible, buy a long term care policy designed to pay a fixed benefit while the insured is in a nursing home. At the least, a policy that pays $80 per day will provide about $29,000 per year.

- A good long term policy should pay if the insured person can't perform certain activities of daily living such as dressing and using the bathroom.

- Severe memory loss, such as dementia or Alzheimer's Disease should qualify a person for benefits.

- Be sure to consider protection against inflation.

- The policy should provide for care in any type of nursing home for at least three years.

- Be aware that Long Term Care policies can be expensive, especially when bought by the elderly. Coverage can cost up to $2000 or more per year for a 60 or 70 year old, double that for a couple. What's more, a 65 year old could end up paying $40,000 in premiums over 20 years and never collect a penny if nursing home care is not necessary.

If the above has you confused, there is an alternative; a life insurance policy that has a special rider which enables the insured to tap a death benefit early, in case of catastrophic illness or long term nursing home costs. Unfortunately, life insurance is more expensive than LTC insurance, but at least someone will collect, as long as you pay the premiums.

Other general considerations to keep in mind when shopping for an insurance policy:

- Don't automatically buy the lowest price policy. It may provide inferior coverage and unaffordable premium increases.

- Try to purchase a comprehensive policy that covers both home care, with a wide range of services, as well as nursing home coverage.

- Be sure to continue coverage provided by employers if you change jobs or if the plan is terminated.

- Avoid policies that require a hospital stay of at least three days before paying nursing home benefits. Thirty-eight states have made that requirement illegal.

- When purchasing a policy for home health care, look for one that pays for aides who help patients with personal or custodial care, rather than one that pays for skilled personnel such as registered nurses.

- Be wary if a policy requires that care be medically necessary for sickness or injury.

- Get the shoppers' guide on long-term care written by the National Association of Insurance Commissioners before you buy. Take time and read it.

In summary, pre-plan as far in advance as you can. Be careful (Caveat Emptor) and shop wisely when purchasing an insurance policy. Remember, the number of people needing nursing home care in the United States alone will triple in the next 40 years.

In addition, write Congress and your legislators. Demand that something be done for individuals who have been taxpayers all their lives, who have been useful members of society and saved for their old age, only to have their life's work and dreams disappear while paying for nursing home care.

Eleven

LEGAL ASPECTS

The great thing in this world is not so much where we are, but in what direction we are moving.

Oliver Wendell Holmes

After the frustration of searching for insurance coverage, you will probably experience another dilemma when you are forced to consider the legal aspects concerned with catastrophic illness. Medicaid pays the bill for the indigent, but the vast majority of citizens or the middle class individuals or families must spend down to a few thousand dollars in order to qualify for such assistance. Most states have laws that allow a surviving spouse to remain in the family home and continue receiving one-half of the couple's assets (Social Security, pensions, etc.). Otherwise, individuals must spend down to a certain level before they qualify for assistance. Faced with long-term nursing home bills, many elderly people are forced to give away all their assets to survive the costs of medical care.

With pre-planning, there are legal ways to protect your assets from the tremendous costs of nursing home care.

Let's look at some of the history of laws dealing with the problem.

In 1981 in California, The Department of Health Services advised Marc Hankin's mother to divorce his father, an Alzheimer's patient and her husband of 45 years, to protect her assets. He was incensed. At the time Mr. Hankins was a first year law student. In 1984, and by then an attorney, he co-sponsored a bill with Assembly woman Jean M. Moorhead (D-Sacramento) which required the health department's MediCal administration to furnish applicants for MediCal funding with a written statement of their rights. This was a step in the right direction but more was needed.

In 1985, also in California, AB 1667, (Chapter 1031, Statutes of 1983) amended state law so that a spouse living at home would be entitled to receive one-half of the couple's income when the other spouse was in a nursing home. Most states have a similar law. The Department of Health Services did not implement the legislation until the court case, Reese vs. Kizer was put into effect. There was still a catch - people who wanted to get the benefit of the new rule would have to ask MediCal workers to divide up their community property income.

Be aware that coverage for nursing home services is limited. The requirements for becoming eligible for assistance varies from state to state. As of January 1, 1989, Medicare pays for the first 150 days of skilled nursing home care in a Medicare-certified skilled nursing home. No benefits are provided for intermediate nursing or custodial care. How many American families can finance a $30,000 to $40,000 a year nursing home care bill when they are over sixty-five or seventy years of age? Not very many. You can contact your local Social Security office or Public Social Services for eligibility requirements for Medicaid. Clearly, federal legislation is needed to alleviate the problems.

In 1990, there were approximately 1,500,000 people in nursing homes, the majority over 80 years of age, mostly middle class. Half of that number have Alzheimer's disease or other dementias. Unless you plan, every single asset you have could be spent paying for long-term care.

Boston attorney, Harley Gordon, author of *How To Protect Your Life Savings From Catastrophic Illness and Nursing Homes*, made several recommendations to older people. One way to protect your assets is to put your house in trust for your children and transfer cash to them. However, all financial transactions must be made 30 months before asking for Medicaid. These guidelines can change.

On a television program produced for Frontline, entitled "Who Pays For Mom and Dad?," over WGBH-TV Boston, MA, and aired on PBS, April 30, 1991, Mr. Gordon discussed three ways to shelter your money: 1) give your assets away; 2) set them up in an irrevocable trust; 3) hold them in joint tenancy. "At some point," he said, "when you have a catastrophe and if you have to go bankrupt, you will have to think about sheltering your money." Pre-planning is advisable. The idea of doing this is to shelter a family's assets somewhere that is legally not counted when a Welfare office is reviewing one's elgibility for Medicaid.

The notion of purposely impoverishing oneself in order to qualify for Medicaid (a form of welfare) sounds to some as very un-American. Jayne Bryant Quinn, an economist and syndicated columnist, has argued against lawyers like Mr. Gordon and says this is an issue not of legality but of fairness.

"We don't have enough money in the states to provide enough home health care, meals on wheels, etc. for the elderly who do not have to go into nursing homes. There are not enough tax dollars out there to help these elderly people, and yet the affluent elderly in a nursing home who have hidden their money suddenly get all the tax dollars."

On the same PBS program, Representative Henry Waxman, Subcommittee on Health and the Environment was interviewed. He said,

"I think that when Medicare was adopted, we were looking at the acute care, the hospitalizations, as the biggest issue and that people wouldn't live much beyond a spell of illness if it got serious enough. We didn't know that we'd have such a graying of the American population. We didn't anticipate the *non system* that we have or the enormous need that we now have for the long-term care for the elderly."

As noted in the Chapter on Insurance, in Charlie's and my case, he qualified for MediCal at one point, but I didn't feel he was ready for a nursing home at that time. I continued to spend my own money to pay for him, money that had always been kept legally separate from his, in trust for my children. In 1990 the law changed in California which forced me to include all assets as community property when considering eligibility for MediCal. Since I no longer owned a home, I was told to spend down to a few thousand dollars in order for Charlie to qualify for MediCal. I found myself in a bind. How would I provide for my own old age.

Attorney Gordon recommends buying long term insurance if you can qualify for and afford a good policy. Unfortunately, most middle class individuals cannot. He does not recommend applying for Medicaid before entering a nursing home. "Many nursing homes don't welcome Medicaid patients because reimbursement rates are so low. Keep some money in your own name. Not only will you preserve independence, you'll be able to enter an excellent nursing home as a private pay patient." He also cautions caregivers not to let parents or a spouse enter a nursing home that is exclusively private-pay if they intend to apply for Medicaid later.

The real dilemma is that neither Medicare nor private insurance companies (with a few expensive exceptions) cover the type of care required for Alzheimer patients. There is a real need for legislation to establish custodial-care policies.

Consider another case discussed on the PBS program. A man (He asked not to be identified) whose wife had Alzheimer's had spent about $60,000 for her care in a nursing home. He went to Mr. Gordon asking advice on how to avoid spending any more. He started out with $125,000 and was told that he would have to spend down to $2000 before his wife could get Medicaid. Mr. Gordon told him that was wrong. This man would not have known that if he had not sought legal advice. In 1991, Medicaid law allowed a spouse to keep half of the family assets up to a limit of $66,480, but the amount changes yearly.

All across America, families of the elderly are looking to the federal government for a program to help pay for middle-class Americans who have to go to nursing homes. In 1989, the Claude Pepper Congressional commission examined issues of financing long -term care. After hearing testimony from many families facing a crisis, it made recommendations, knowing that the government must play a role. The Pepper Commission's proposals take Medicare, state monies, insurance policies, and individual payments into account, but will be expensive to implement.

At present, in the absence of any legislation to help individuals pay for long term care, the goal, according to recommendations by Mr. Gordon, is to remain independent and self-supporting as long as possible. When all else fails, then consider Medicaid qualification. One of the fastest growing legal specialties that covers the entire spectrum of legal issues facing older Americans is "Elder Law." David Averbuck, a consulting attorney for the Family Survival Project of San Francisco says, "Elder Law is all about control and empowerment." Blending the legal tools of wills, trust, and convservatorships with a heavy dose of preventive planning is necessary. Consider the following case.

Mrs. Jones, whose husband had developed Alzheimer's Disease, but was still competent, was told by attorneys there was nothing she could do to plan for their estate. She was warned not to give away any assets because that would be defrauding the government. Luckily she didn't give up. When attending a meeting of the Alzheimer's Disease and Related Disorders Association (ADRDA) in her community, she learned that there were many steps she and her husband could follow to plan for the future. Those suggestions could apply to anyone planning an estate.

- Sign durable powers of attorney incorporating specific and sophisticated powers necessary for public benefits planning.

- Put the family home exclusively in the caregiving spouse or child's name so the ill person will become eligible for Medicaid (MediccCal in California) benefits and the home can be secured for the spouse and/or the children.

- Divest yourself of certain assets and contractually divide community property assets to get maximum benefit from eligibility rules.

- Execute a revocable trust agreement that incorporates Medicaid (MediCal) planning options and avoids probate and the need for a conservatorship.

- Execute durable powers of attorney for health care to make sure that a conservator will not be necessary for this purpose.

By the year 2000, the price tag for health care in America is predicted to be $1.5 trillion — $5,550 per person or approximately 15% of our gross national product. Our $2,425 per individual cost at present is 38% more than

Canada, twice what Japan pays and almost three times what Great Britain pays. The problem isn't the amount of money we invest, it is in our health care delivery system itself, which is too fragmented.

It is estimated that the number of people needing nursing home care in the United States alone will triple in the next 40 years. It is essential that a decision be made on what it is we want for the elderly. The federal government must be involved, as well as the state governments. Private insurers and families all must take some responsibility if we are to implement a viable health care plan for elderly citizens.

Notes

Twelve

HOPE FOR THE FUTURE

Hope springs eternal in the human breast.

Alexander Pope

When dealing with this debilitating disease, you may feel all is hopeless. Watching a loved one slowly deteriorate, diminish, and disappear before your eyes can be very depressing. Is there any hope for the future? Yes, there is. Researchers all over the world are working on problems of the aging, dementia, and especially Alzheimer's Disease.

I remember the dread in many hearts when epidemics of polio, smallpox, typhoid, and diphtheria decimated the population. Now those illnesses and many others are controlled, due mainly to the dedicated men and women who discovered cures.

More than 80 years after the German neurologist, Alois Alzheimer, discovered damaged cells in the brain of a demented patient, the mind-killing condition remains a great medical mystery. Many researchers are busy trying to link it to genes, to infections, to toxic agents, or to flaws in the machinery by which the cells build and break down vital chemicals. But so far no one can say yet what causes Alzheimer's disease or even how it does its damage. No one yet knows how to prevent or cure it.

Physicians often have a difficult time diagnosing this disease which starts with memory loss. After a thorough checkup that will exclude other ailments, doctors assume that the patient has Alzheimer's, although only an autopsy will give a positive diagnosis. Alzheimer's often goes undiagnosed because of a tendency to attribute early symptoms to the normal effects of aging.

In recent years, the accuracy of Alzheimer's diagnosis has improved up to 90 percent. Through research and clinical studies, medical experts now agree on standardized criteria for diagnosis.

Clinical studies also have resulted in the use of new technology to diagnose Alzheimer's. An MRI (magnetic resonance imaging) scan uses magnetic beams to give a sharp, detailed picture of brain tissue, and a PET (positron emission tomography) scan identifies areas of the brain where abnormal activity is present.

WHAT IS BEING DONE?

The founding President of the Alzheimer's Disease and Related Disorders Association (ADRDA), Jerome H. Stone, made it the first priority of the group to research into finding the cause, treatment, and cure for Alzheimer's Disease. Education about the disease for general practitioners, nursing practitioners, home caregivers, and the public will take high priority.

Scientists state that previously Alzheimer's was thought of as senility, but in fact it's been around for thousands of years. Peter Rabins, M.D., Johns Hopkins School of Medicine says, "I think what we have learned in the last 15 or 20 years is that, in fact, it is a disease, or a group of diseases, and not normal aging."

In 1987, The National Institute of Aging announced that it would spend $2 million a year to study an experimental drug called THA or Tracine (tetrahydroaminocridine), one of the first drugs ever alleged to reverse memory loss due to Alzheimer's. Because very sophisticated monitoring is required to successfully administer the drug, only a few medical centers in the United States can utilize procedures which are deemed necessary. The Food and Drug Administration requested that the study be stopped after some of the patients displayed serious side effects, including liver toxicity, but this doesn't mean that we shouldn't keep on trying. A new set of clinical trials has been called for to give clear evidence of the drug's effectiveness.

In 1987, Dorothy Kirsten French, the former Metropolitan diva, opened the John Douglas French Center in Los Alamitos, California, as a tribute to her spouse. Her husband, world-renowned neurosurgeon, John Douglas French, had been diagnosed with Alzheimer's. At first, Mrs. French brought in around-the-clock nursing assistance, trying to care for him in their home. Eventually it became dangerous for him to remain at home. The French Alzheimer's Center now sponsors public service seminars and Mrs. French has stated, "Because we feel that we are on the edge of finding that first breakthrough, I am determined that the John Douglas French Foundation find it. We have gatherings of the finest scientists we can find, not only in our country but in the world." Encouraging words.

Many other individuals not in the field of science are also engaged in the battle to find a cure for Alzheimer's. There are countless volunteer supports nationwide. Many companies have become involved. For example, Home Savings of America has contributed over $400,000, which has been used principally to help ADRDA chapters around the country in their fundraising efforts.

In responding to the request for funds to study the disease, Congressman Edward Roybal of the House Select Committee on Aging, urged that new legislation be passed. "The committee on appropriations was able to make the first proposal for $5 million dollars. We now have $50 million, but the truth of the matter is that we need $500 million . . .We, as a nation, are not responding to this epidemic with new legislation. The people can bring about a change by writing letters, making telephone calls, talking to their representatives, and letting them know that they want changes in the entire field of health, and that one place to start is with funding more money for basic research." You can start your own letter writing campaign and help ensure that new legislation is passed.

In 1990, Dr. Frederick Bonte and his colleagues at the University of Texas Southwestern Medical Center in Dallas announced a new approach to help diagnose Alzheimer's, previously one of the most frustrating aspects of the disease. Using a computer enhanced scanner technique called SPECT they can trace a radioactive substance through body tissue. Doctors can now look inside a living patient's brain. Using a chemical that settles in brain tissues in direct proportion to the amount of blood flow in that area, doctors can identify abnormalities in the brain's blood flow that point to Alzheimer's.

Over the last ten to fifteen years, researchers have begun to unravel the secrets of physiological events responsible for the destruction of brain cells that marks Alzheimer's disease. It is now recognized that the disease takes several forms: one that strikes before age 55 and runs in families, another appears after the age of 65. In both types, two proteins that are somehow involved in the death of nerve cells essential to memory, emotions, and thought are involved. Evidence supporting a genetic defect in one of those proteins was compelling. Now two laboratories have announced the creation of genetically engineered mice that carry copies of the human gene for the protein for research purposes.

DRUG RESEARCH

The Federal Drug Administration (FDA) has raised drugs used to treat Alzheimer's to the same level of urgency as treatments for cancer and AIDS. "The drugs should be pushed ahead as fast as possible, but high scientific standards must be kept at the same time," said FDA Commissioner David Kessler. "Sadly, the experimental drugs available for Alzheimer's are limited." This is a giant step, offering some hope to those now suffering from Alzheimer's.

According to a report released by ADRDA and the pharmaceutical companies researching possible drugs, the first medicines expected to become available in 1991, although not a cure, do represent important progress toward easing the symptoms of the disease.

A simple test, developed at the University of Minnesota in 1989 to help Alzheimer's patients in early stages of brain disorder, has won praise from the American Medical Association. The 10-word memory test, which takes less than 10 minutes, seems to be an accurate means of predicting Alzheimer's, according to the American Medical Association.

Thus far, only a handful of drugs have shown promise. THA or Tracine, which slows the natural breakdown of acetylcholine is only of temporary value to few patients. Another drug, desferrioxamine, thought to neutralize aluminum, proved unhelpful after a two year study. Currently, more promise is sought by researchers studying nerve growth faction, a naturally occurring protein that coddles and replenishes nerve cells. It has been found to work on animals on the very same cells that suffer the most in human brains with Alzheimer's disease.

MORE RESEARCH

The Alzheimer's Disease Research Center at the University of California, Irvine, recently became one of the nine state-sponsored AD Diagnostic and Treatment Centers and is the Orange County Branch of the federally-sponsored Southern California Alzheimer's research consortiums.

James L. McGaugh, Ph.D., psychobiologist and former vice-chancellor of the University, is one researcher who is actively involved in this area. Being his assistant in the late 1960s, when he was Dean of the School of Biological Sciences, opened up a wonderful new world for me. A visit in the fall of 1990 to his office and to the office of Carl Cotman, Ph.D., Director of the Center, provided me with a gold-mine of information on advances in the field.

The Alzheimer's Research Center's May, 1990 bulletin stated that preliminary results from a new program at the University of California, Irvine, show that 'memory repair' may be possible for those in the early stages of Alzheimer's disease. Drs. Curt Sandman, Patrick Kesslak, and Karen Nackoul are developing an AD memory training program that not only identifies patients' cognitive strengths and weaknesses, but also provides them with the means to help compensate for their losses. The University of California Irvine (UCI) Memory Training Program runs for eight consecutive weeks (four weeks of training and four weeks of support group) and is offered by ADDTC four to five times yearly. Caregivers and patients must participate. Only select patients are eligible since the program does not appear helpful for late-stage Alzheimer's patients.

Several researchers have said that trying to understand the disease is like working on a puzzle in a roomful of pieces that may not fit. But sixteen medicines are being developed by eleven pharmaceutical companies to treat the disease and its related symptoms.

Genetics

Considerable research has focused on whether heredity has a part in causing Alzheimer's. Family members of most persons with Alzheimer's have only a slightly increased chance of developing the disease over that of other individuals. However, the risk is much greater when a family member develops the disease before age 50. Scientists have established that an inherited form of Alzheimer's definitely exists in the families of younger Alzheimer's patients. Recently, a study tracing the inherited form within a family in Indiana was announced.

Heredity is determined by biological material known as KNA. This is contained in genes which are located on chromosomes. In paricular, genetic research is concentrating on chromosome 21. Scientists believe that chromosome 21 plays a significant role in the development of Alzheimer's because of the connection between Alzheimer's and Down's syndrome.

Down's syndrome (mongolism) results in mental retardation and other birth defects. People with Down's syndrome have an extra chromosome 21. If they survive into middle age, these individuals frequently develop changes in the brain that are identical to those in Alzhimer's. The similarities between premature aging of the brain in Down's syndrome patients and the Alzheimer's brain have been the basis of several important research effortss.

Scientists found that chromosome 21 does contain at least one gene responsible for the inherited form of Alzheimer's. Recent studies also show that the gene which manufactures amyloid (protein fragments) is located on chromosome 21.

Donald Price, a neurobiologist at Johns Hopkins, believes that the research on beta amyloid in the brains of Alzheimer's patients will be enhanced when studies of the tangles inside dying neurons can be made. They have barely been able to unravel this mystery in laboratories because the neurons are almost impossible to dissolve.

British researchers have reported that they have identified a possible genetic cause of Alzheimer's. Researchers at St. Mary's Hospital Medical School in London studied two families prone to the disease; they found a genetic mutation that alters a protein present in large quantities in the brains of people with Alzheimer's.

Findings published in Proceedings of the National Academy of Sciences state that researchers involved in a recent series of studies have come close to identifying the precise cause of the disorder and are developing new theories. Neurologist Creighton Phelps of the Alzheimer's Association said, "We're getting right to the heart of the matter, that beta-amyloid seems to be playing a very key role in Alzheimer's. We can't say it's the cause quite yet, but if we can block it, we may very well be able to slow down or stop the progression of the disease."

At Boston's Childrens' Hospital, Neurologist Bruce Yanker said that members of the team are already studying the effects of the brain hormone, called substance P, in other animals, including primates, and that they could possibly begin studying the material in humans within five years.

Relief cannot come quickly enough for families of Alzheimer's Disease patients. Patricia Huebner, whose mother-in-law, Alice Zilonka, has the disease and whose story was covered in U.S. News and World Reports Magazine in August, 1991, said, "This disease doesn't destroy the person: they don't know what's going on. Alzheimer's destroys the family."

SUMMARY

I will continue to care for my Charlie, encouraged by reports of all the dedicated, intelligent scientists, doctors, nurses, biologists, and others who are working on a greater understanding of this terrible disease. I remind myself that research takes time and treatment that would help Charlie may never occur in his lifetime. Nevertheless, I am optimistic. I feel sparks of hope when I realize that all over the world there are people who care.

Taking care of an Alzheimer patient is called the 36-hour day for good reason. As one victim's husband wrote to the Alzheimer's Family Relief Program, "It's like caring for a 150 pound infant who needs constant attention...an infant who asks you the same question 50 times a day...an infant who will never grow up...there's no peace...no time to rest."

Coping Strategies

I have thought a lot about how I managed to cope, and about the coping methods I have heard or read about which helped me during the last few years. Remember, however, that what works for one Alzheimer's patient may not work for another. For example, it was most difficult for me to learn patience as I had been an impatient person all of my life. No matter how hard I tried, I was not always patient with Charlie. Many times I would rush into our bedroom, bury my head in a pillow, and scream. I learned that you can have all kinds of thoughts and feelings toward the patient, such as anger, resentment, and guilt, because sometimes you feel that your loved one might be better off if he died. But it's best to think positively as much as possible. Remember that you are not alone. There are many caregivers in the same situation.

Find a support group. The Alzheimer's Association has to date over 200 Chapters nationwide that offer family members referrals to helpful services in their communities. Several European countries also have Chapters. These Association Chapters sponsor family support groups that give family members a chance to share their experiences and learn new techniques for coping with Alzheimer's.

In the day-to-day routine it is important to adapt to the needs of your patient and to be sensitive to his changing moods, avoiding situations that trigger unwanted reactions. If he does become belligerent, be quiet, nod agreement even if you have to lie a bit to soothe his belligerency. Try to move slowly and use a calm voice so as not to add to his tension. Listen well as good listening can be a de-escalator of tension. Listen, even when his words are incoherent and hard to understand. Encourage him to talk, and always speak face-to-face with him, never from behind. Do not discuss his condition with others within his hearing range. Do not ask questions that test the patient's memory. Sit close to him and touch him. The pressure of your hand during moments of silence can communicate support and love. Affection can often defuse a difficult situation.

As stated previously, don't be afraid that Alzheimer's is catching. There is no evidence that it can be passed from one person to another. The exception is an inheritance factor, which some researchers estimate to be 30 percent. You may have days when you feel you also have Alzheimer's. When I can't remember something I feel I should, I ask myself, "Am I developing the disease?" Then I calm myself down by considering that I acted the same way when I was much younger. I recall someone saying, "If you can't find your keys, you're OK. But if you have the keys in your hand and don't know what to do with them, you have a dementia problem."

Perhaps the following acronym will help you keep some other pointers in mind:

ALZHEIMER'S COPING ACRONYM

A for   **ACCEPTANCE** as opposed to resignation. Acceptance is an act of the will; a commitment to finding resources within yourself to get through denial and guilt, to believe in yourself and be kind to yourself.

L for   **LISTENING and LAUGHTER.** Be a good listener even when his or her words are incoherent and hard to understand. Watch TV together. Select programs for their humor.

Z for   **ZEST.** These coping strategies will help you keep your zest for living despite all you're going through.

H for   **HOME SAFETY FEATURES.** Follow some of the suggestions in Chapter Eight to help keep your loved one safe while caring for him at home. Several were of great assistance to me when Charlie was still at home.

E for   **EDUCATION.** Keep informed about pending legislation and current research. Knowledge is empowering.

I for   **INVOLVEMENT.** Don't try to carry the whole burden yourself. Seek help from relatives, friends, and community services. Take time off if possible. Get involved in a support group. It really helps.

M for	**MEDITATION and PRAYER.** Don't give up even though your prayers aren't answered. Pray for patience, pray for understanding; pray for your Alzheimer's patient.
E for	**EMPATHY and ENCOURAGEMENT.** Encourage your loved one to talk even when it is boring for you. It is important that his dignity be preserved, and he be helped to feel worthwhile by encouraging him/her to participate in as many activities and duties as he is capable of.
R for	**RECOGNITION.** It is difficult to face the reality that the person you once loved is no longer the person you once knew, but the only way to make peace with your situation in the long run.
S for	**SELF CARE.** Just as in an airplane we are instructed to put on our own oxygen mask before assisting a child with hers, so you must take care of yourself in order to be able to care for your loved one.

I hope that in the sharing of our story, I have offered you some helpful ideas. I urge you to consider the options. Pre-plan for your insurance and financial needs. Become familiar with the legal aspects involved, and plan your estate with this in mind. Start a letter writing campaign to Congress asking for new legislation and better health coverage for all.

PART III

RESOURCES

Resources

CAREGIVER BILL OF RIGHTS *

Inasmuch as WE, THE CAREGIVERS, devote ourselves and our internal and external resources to the maintenance and support of a loved one, we declare that we have basic inalienable rights. Furthermore, we recognize that we are not alone in our challenge to maintain a humane lifestyle for ourselves and our loved ones; therefore, we pledge our support to all who struggle with balancing the responsibilities of daily living. With this in mind we mandate the following rights:

- The Right To Live Our Own Life And Retain Our Dignity And Sense Of Self.

- The Right To Choose A Plan Of Caring That Accommodates Our Needs And The Needs Of Those We Care About.

- The Right To Be Recognized As A Vital And Stabilizing Source Within Our Families.

- The Right To Be Free Of Guilt, Anguish, And Doubt Knowing That The Decisions We Make Are Appropriate For Our Own Well-being And That Of Our Loved One.

- The Right To Be Ourselves Enough To Have Confidence That We Are Doing The Best That We Are Able.

With these rights, the disabled and frail elderly will be provided the highest and best care that we are capable of giving, and we may take pride in ourselves.

* Source Unknown

ORGANIZATIONS

Alzheimer's Disease and Related Disorders Associates, Inc. (ADRDA)
919 N. Michigan Ave., Suite 1000
Chicago, IL. 60611-1676
(800) 272-3900.   CA only (800) 660-1993

American Association of Retired Persons (AARP),
1909 K Street, N.W.,
Washington, D.C. 20049.
(800) 245-1212 Group Health Insurance

The American Association of Retired Persons will provide the following free publications:
> Making Wise Decisions for Long Term Care (D12435): A guide to long term care services and financing.
>
> A Path for Caregivers (D12957): A guide for individuals with caregiving identifying both national and local resources.
>
> Nursing Home Life: A Guide to Long Term Care Insurance (D12893): Provides tips on evaluating the need for long term care insurance as well as on comparing policies.

Burke Rehabilitation Hospital,
Community Relations Department,
785 Mamaroneck Avenue,
White Plains, New York 10605
(914) 948-0050 ext. 2466

Family Survival Project for Brain-Damaged Adults,
1736 Divisidero,
San Francisco, CA 94115

American Society on Aging
833 Market St., Suite 512
San Francisco, CA 94103
(415) 882-2910

National Association for Homecare,
519 C Street, N.E.,
Washington, DC 20002

Partners in Care,
345 Park Avenue, S.,
New York, NY 10160

Support Groups—family, relatives, friends, and local support groups, obtained from telephone books, Chambers of Commerce, and libraries

Visiting Nurses' Service (VNS) Home Care,
107 East 70th Street,
New York, NY 10021
A nonprofit subsidiary of Visiting Nurses Service of New York

SELECTED REFERENCES

Bausell, Ph.D., et al. 1988. *How To Evaluate And Select A Nursing Home*. Reading, MA: Addison-Wesley Publishing Company, Inc.

Begmagin, V. and K. Hirn. 1979. *Aging Is A Family Affair*. New York, NY: Thomas Y.Crowell

Benhamin, Ben. 1981. *Are You Tense?* New York, NY: Pantheon Books

Bernheim, Kayla F., et al. 1982. *The Caring Family—living With Chronic Mental Illness*. New York, NY: Random House

Burger, Sarah Greene and Martha D'Erasmo. 1976. *Living In A Nursing Home*. New York: Ballantine Books

Burke Rehabilitation Center. 1991. *Home Management of the Person with Intellectual Loss (Dementia or Alzheimer's Disease)*. White Plains, NY 10605

Burke Rehabilitation Center. 1989. *Choosing a Nursing Home for the Person with Intellectural Loss,* White Plains, NY 10605

Einsdorfer, Carl, Ph.D. and Donna Cohen, Ph.D. *Management of the Patient and Family Coping With Dementing Illness*. Journal of Family Practice 12, no. 5, 1981: 831-837

Felder, Leonard, Ph.D. 1990. *When A Loved One Is Ill— How To Take Better Care of Your Loved One, Your Family, and Yourself.* New York, NY: New American Library, a Division of Penguin Books, USA Inc.

Glascote, R. and Gudeman, Jr. 1977. *Creative Mental Health Services For The Elderly.* Washington, DC: The Joint Information Service.

Horne, Jo. 1989. *The Nursing Home Handbook*. Glenview, IL: AARP and Scott, Foresman and Company

Institute on Law and Rights of Older Adults, *The Medicaid Program.* New York, NY: Brookdale Center on Aging of Hunter College, 1981

Kenny, James and S. Spicer. 1984. *Caring For Your Aging Parents: A Practical Guide To The Challenges, The Choices*. Cincinnati, OH: St. Anthony Messenger Press

Klipper, Miriam. 1975. *The Relaxation Response*. New York, NY: Avon Books

Mace, Nancy L. and Peter V. Rabins, M.D. 1981. *The 36-Hour Day—A Family Guide to Caring For Persons With Alzheimer's Disease, Related Dementing Illnesses, And Memory Loss in Later Life*. Baltimore: Johns Hopkins University University Press

McGaugh, James L., Ph.D. *Significance and Remembrance: The Role of Neuromodulatory Systems*. Psychological Science 1990 vol. no. 1, pp 15-25

National Council on the Aging, 1982. *Adult Day Care*. Annotated Bibliography. Washington, DC

National Foundation for Medical Research, Guy Luskin. 1990. *The Living Death: Alzheimer's in America*. Washington, D.C.: Potomac Publishing Company

Parker, C.M. 1972. *Bereavement Studies Of Grief In Adult Life*. London: Tavistock Institute of Human Relations

Prudden, Bonnie. 1960. *Keep Fit, Be Happy*. Warner Bros. Records, Inc. (B-1358)

Springer, Dianne and Timothy Brubaker. 1981. *Family Caregiving And Dependent Elderly*. Beverly Hills, CA: Sage Publications, Inc.

Watkins, Donald M. 1983. *Handbook Of Nutrition, Health And Aging*. Park Ridge, NJ: Noyes Publications

Resources

INDEX

ORDER FORM

Pathfinder Publishing of California
458 Dorothy Ave.
Ventura, CA 93003
Telephone (805) 642-9278   FAX (805) 650-3656

Please send me the following books from Pathfinder Publishing:

_____Copies of **Agony & Death on a**
             Gold Rush Steamer @ $8.95 $_____
_____Copies of **Beyond Sympathy** @ $9.95 $_____
_____Copies of **Dialogues In Swing** @ $12.95 $_____
_____Copies of **Final Celebrations** @ $9.95 $_____
_____Copies of **Let Your Ideas Speak Out** @ $8.95 $_____
_____Copies of **Life With Charlie** @ $9.95 $_____
_____Copies of **Living Creatively**
             With Chronic Illness @ $11.95 $_____
_____Copies of **More Dialogues In Swing**
             Softcover @ $14.95 $_____
             Hardcover @ $22.95 $_____
_____Copies of **No Time For Goodbyes** @ $9.95 $_____
_____Copies of **Quest For Respect** @ $7.95 $_____
_____Copies of **Stop Justice Abuse** @ $10.95 $_____
_____Copies of **Surviving a Japanese POW Camp**
             @ $11.95 $_____
_____Copies of **Shipwrecks, Smugglers & Maritime**
Mysteries @ $9.95 $_____
_____Copies of **World of Gene Krupa** @ $14.95 $_____
                          Sub-Total $_____
      Californians: Please add 7.25% tax. $_____
      Shipping* $_____
                     Grand Total $_____

I understand that I may return the book for a full refund if not satisfied.
Name:_____

Address:_____
_____ZIP:_____

*SHIPPING CHARGES U.S.
Books: Enclose $2.50 for the first book and .50c for each additional book. UPS: Truck; $3.50 for first item, .50c for each additional. UPS Air: $5.00 for first item, $1.50 for each additional item.